BYPASS

BYPASS

A Doctor's Recovery from Open Heart Surgery

by
JOSEPH D. WAXBERG, M.D.

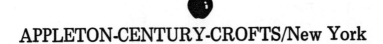

APPLETON-CENTURY-CROFTS/New York

Copyright © 1981 by APPLETON-CENTURY-CROFTS
A Publishing Division of Prentice-Hall, Inc.

81 82 83 84 85 / 10 9 8 7 6 5 4 3 2 1

Prentice-Hall International, Inc., London
Prentice-Hall of Australia, Pty. Ltd., Sydney
Prentice-Hall of India Private Limited, New Delhi
Prentice-Hall of Japan, Inc., Tokyo
Prentice-Hall of Southeast Asia (Pte.) Ltd., Singapore
Whitehall Books Ltd., Wellington, New Zealand

Library of Congress Cataloging in Publication Data

Waxberg, Joseph D., 1922–
  Bypass, a doctor's recovery from open heart surgery.

  1. Heart—Surgery—Patients—United States—Biography.
2. Physicians—United States—Biography. 3. Waxberg,
Joseph D., 1922–   . I. Title.
RD598.W33   617'.412   81-12882
ISBN 0-8385-0935-5   AACR2

Text design: Judith Warm-Steinig
Cover design: Gloria J. Moyer
Production Editor: Ina Shapiro

PRINTED IN THE UNITED STATES OF AMERICA

To my family
Carol
Anita and Jonathan
Charles
"Nana"
Thelma Harris

Contents

BYPASS

One

The First Symptoms

It was a Thursday evening, a little after 11:00, and we were in bed. Carol and I were watching the news on television. It was December 15 and we were talking about our two boys coming home for Christmas.

While we were talking, I began to have this vague feeling in my abdomen and chest. It was the first pain — no, not pain: the first unfamiliar feeling that came across my chest, a pressure, a something I had never felt before.

One recognizes signs and symptoms, aches and strains and pains, a multitude of physical changes too varied to mention. A gastric colic, indigestion, and nausea all have to do with the same area, and yet each indicates to the brain the differences among the three of them. Although they share an obvious similiarity, pink, red, and crimson are distinct colors. So, too, there are at least as many messages of physical distress as there are organs in one's body. I know, in fact, there are very many feelings and symptoms associated with each of these organs, but this pressure in my chest was totally unfamiliar. It was not pink or red or crimson. I tolerated the discomfort in a detached way; I suspect that detachment had become a habit after a quarter

century as an introspective physician, a psychiatrist. It is important to be aware of this so that you can understand the feelings
and thoughts that raced (but always in one conscious direction)
through my mind: I was determined to be true to myself, not
to lie, because the end result is that you become a foolish
liar, which is not the sort of person I would be interested in
knowing.

So, detached, I waited that evening for the symptoms to
change, perhaps to change to something more familiar, a little
more on the pink side or a little more on the red side, even a
little more on the crimson side. This strange conglomerate hue,
this tint with which I was totally unfamiliar, I had difficulty in
coping with this.

I had been married more than 20 years to the same woman
whom I had met when I was in psychiatric residency, someone
who has always been very special, someone whose intuition I
could depend upon in dealing with someone like myself. I made
no mention of my feelings and thoughts as we sat there that
evening. At 55 years of age, fairly athletic, never ill (aside from
ordinary colds and an occasional flu), the thought of some coronary problem was distant from my psychic conscious mechanism. Yet, as remote as I thought it was, the word was, as one
would say, on the "tip of my tongue." I felt that if I did not use
the word or bring it up in conversation with Carol, the symptoms would change their color and become recognizable as a tint
with which I was more familiar.

After a half hour, the symptoms pointed like arrows at the
bull's eye of my mind. I felt concerned for Carol. How would I
tell her without arousing excessive fear? It could have been
nothing: some strange symptoms of indigestion or a hiatal her-
nia that had poked itself into existence in recent months. My
concern was with the way to relay the necessity of both of us
getting into the car and of her driving me to the emergency
room at the hospital. The pressure persisted, refused to be distracted, and now I was becoming apprehensive.

Finally, I said, "I think we should go to the emergency room
at the hospital." I can still remember her face. We had been
chatting about our two boys. A great pride and joy to us, the

elder was in his second year at medical school, and the younger was completing college. Her pleasant, attractive face meant so much to me. I would have given a diamond to prevent cause for a tear in the corner of her eye. We began to dress; as I removed my pajamas, the discomfort began to subside and then to disappear.

"This is nonsense," I said. "Forget it. Let's get back to bed."

"Are you certain?" Carol asked.

"Yes." We returned to bed.

I turned on the TV to distract my attention. Little by little, that annoying pressure returned. I hesitated again to say anything, but in the glow from the TV set I could see Carol watching me, alert for my reactions. Finally, "I think we should go," I said. "This feeling is coming back."

Again we dressed and I asked Carol to drive. "Are you all right?" she asked as we headed for the hospital.

"I'm not sure," I said candidly. "As a physician I'm aware that the pressure in my chest may be a sign of a coronary."

At this point she drove through a red light, then the next red light and all the others. I sat back trying to remain calm, my thoughts racing. Fear, a symptom not part of my character, began to overwhelm me. I kept these thoughts to myself. My father died of a coronary when he was quite young, and my mother died of a coronary, too: genetically, I was predisposed to a coronary infarct.

The emergency room of Stamford Hospital was bustling: There were three severe burn cases, a knifing, and a mauling by an icepick making a mockery of the human body. The respect for my teaching and concern for humanity lay about me, taunting me. I felt guilt about taking a bed and taking up my fellow physicians' time for an as yet undiagnosed chest job.

Then just as suddenly as it appeared, the pressure in my chest disappeared. It was like a toothache that no longer hurts when one enters the dentist's waiting room.

The chief nurse, Terry Durling, approached. "I don't remember calling you," she said. She assumed I was there to see a patient requiring psychiatric consultation.

"I had some chest pain," I answered, emphasizing the word
had.

With one intense glance at my face she said, "This way,
Doctor," and led me to the cardiac room off to one side of the
emergency department. I removed my pants and shirt and got
into the bed. When Carol was noticed by the nurse, I introduced
her as my wife. I could imagine Terry's thoughts: Should she ask
Carol to wait outside? But she said nothing and left the room. In
seconds she returned with a young resident in internal medicine.

Blood was drawn. An EKG was done; the strong snake-like
wires were whipped to my arms, legs, and chest. Cardiologists
appeared, as did my dear friend Donald Kanter, an internist.
There was movement and scurrying and whispering, and with
each moment my anxiety heightened. You see, if one is going to
have a severe coronary, there is always a possibility that one's
last moment on this earth could be frighteningly close. My good
friend Don reappeared and informed me that the electrocardiogram had indicated some ischemia.

That was the verdict, ischemia. What is this word, *ischemia?* I
deal in different words: *unconscious, dream material, wishes,
guilt, fears, realities* and even *unrealities*. We are both physicians, but we deal with completely separate languages. He says
ischemia. I know what it means: a diminished amount of blood
supply or oxygen to an area, in this case, I suppose, to my heart
muscle. I also know that diminished oxygen to the heart muscle
can produce pain, and it is the earliest sign of some possible
threat to the heart tissue. This is a word that we do not share as
a common source of reference, but I accept it because it is becoming part of my vocabulary.

I question myself. How dare I take a physician from the
havoc in this emergency room, from the cries of the burned
patients searching for relief? I felt for those terribly, painfully
burned men as their voices reached my ears.

Something happens to one's soul when one is strapped to an
EKG machine. The oscilloscope beeps a ceaselessly repeated
tone as it emits waves of green light across the screen, each wave
drifting into silence at the end of the screen. Then the entire
process begins again, over and over, again and again, until time
melts into beeps and lights, and the silence is filled with one's

thoughts. At this point, thoughts are dangerous. This is how it must be for most of us, I think. These are thoughts, surrounded by dreadful sounds.

Don saw that I looked puzzled, but he did not read me too well at that moment. I was feeling extremely apprehensive. "Can you explain this a bit more to me?" I asked. He showed me the EKG. "It's Greek to me," I admitted, looking at the squiggly lines.

"Here," he pointed, "is the S-T wave. It's depressed. It should be a little higher on this reading. It means some part of your heart muscle is not receiving enough blood supply, which carries oxygen to the muscle."

"The pain?" I asked.

"Yes, that causes the pain. At present, we don't know how, or even whether any muscle is involved, but we do know that the blood supply is diminished."

"I feel fine, now," I said. "Does the EKG still show changes?"

"Afraid so," he said. "So we're going to watch you awhile. Frankly, so far, Joe, I think everything is going fairly well. Rest now and be patient with yourself and me. I'll see you again in the morning."

"One more question, Don," I said, glancing at Carol, who was absorbing our conversation. "The nurse gave me Isordel; what is it?"

"It's a medication that decreases the workload of the heart and prevents further ischemia. Any more questions?"

I smiled back. "I'm most appreciative of what you've done, helping me understand what's going on." Actually, I wasn't quite sure of what he had said at that moment. I became apologetic, like a child, and asked: "Am I being a pest?"

"No," he answered, "not yet." He laughed, patted my shoulder and left the room.

It was now time to move me. I was no longer suitable for the emergency room treatment; I was going into the coronary care unit. The bed was wheeled out of the emergency room; there was a bottle of intravenous glucose hanging from a pole, dripping into a vein of my wrist, and I amused myself, my head straight up towards the ceiling, counting the little patches of lights and panels of ceiling tile that were passing by. My eyes became the camera of a grade B movie. The lights passed by rhythmically, without end, a purgatory of movement. Then silence, followed by darkness. And then something new: injections. Through the tubing that was dripping glucose into my vein, a blessed sleeping potion began to mingle with my blood. I could still see the green oscilloscope line waving and winking at me as it ran from the right- to the left-hand corner and then reappeared and repeated its progression. A most damnable invention. Now the strange feeling left — I repeat, it was pressure, not pain — and I finally fell into a restful sleep.

The following morning, Don Kanter arrived with Dr. Richard Landesman, the cardiologist. Richard was friendly, casually dressed, wearing horn-rimmed glasses, and was serious in a professional manner, but pleasant. No alarmist, he. Don excused himself and left Richard to speak to me alone.

Explanations were now necessary. He began to use the language of cardiology. *Ischemia* — remember that word? It had to be caused by something, even though the EKG was normal that morning. Perhaps the amount of ischemia was minimal, or it did not last long enough.

What was he saying to me? He was saying questions to me: not telling me or answering me, *but telling me questions.* We must find out the cause of this ischemia. I asked again, "If the EKG is normal, why do I have to stay here in the coronary care unit?"

"It's not as simple as you think," Richard answered. "The blood supply that we took throughout the evening was tested for enzymes, and this morning, happily, I can tell you that the enzymes are normal."

"What enzymes?" I asked. I was thinking, since the EKG and enzymes are normal, what *is* going on?

"The CPK enzymes," Richard answered.

I nodded. "What does that mean?" I asked.

"Well, that means creatin phosphokinase. The level was 36 last night and the several samples taken during the night were all within normal limits."

"Strange," I thought. "I don't remember them taking blood during the night. Was I that knocked out?" Then I realized all they had to do was to remove the intravenous tubing from the needle, draw a specimen of blood and return the tubing to the needle. Simple — and I'd slept through it all. "What is the abnormal number in the CPK?" I asked.

"About 100," he said. "You were still well below that figure."

Richard pulled a stethoscope from his coat pocket and placed the bell on my chest and listened, first over my left side, then moving it from position to position, listening intently to the sounds. Then he checked my lungs, hearing me breathe in and out. "You must stop smoking," he said quietly.

I said nothing. Stop smoking. How about, "You must climb Mt. Everest!"

When he finished the examination, he said: "We'll watch what happens for a day or two. Everything seems fine."

"Tell me, Richard," I said. "If the EKG is normal and the enzymes are normal, again, why do I have to stay in the hospital?"

"That's what I was hoping you would be curious about, Joe," he said. "If there is an EKG change, regardless of what the enzymes show, there has to be a cause for it."

"Could I have been perhaps tense or distressed about something?" I asked.

"No," he answered. "The EKG simply records the electrical impulses that spread throughout the heart muscle that make it contract. If there is any change in this picture, there has to be a reason for that change, even if it only lasted a few hours during last night. It's your body's way of telling you — informing you, really — that something is awry. I don't know what it is at the moment and I cannot answer your question, but there is a way we can determine the cause of it."

I remember staring at him as he sat at the foot of the bed, talking in his friendly manner to me. There was something about his mannerisms that I liked. He was calm and reassuring; he was also teaching and explaining, and he was not force-feeding me and demanding that I accept his decisions. I appreciated that approach.

"What do we do next?" I asked.

"Well," Richard began, "the only certain way that we

can tell what is going on inside your heart is by doing an
arteriogram."

My brow wrinkled in puzzlement.

"It's rather simple," he explained. "We insert a catheter that
goes into the brachial artery here." He pointed to the inside of
my elbow. "We put the catheter into your brachial artery, as I
said, and then into your subclavian, which goes directly into the
aorta and then into the chambers of the heart. With this catheter
we can measure the volume and the pressure and the flow of
blood through the chambers of your heart. And then we can insert the tip of the catheter into the openings of the various
coronary arteries, and each time inject a small amount of dye,
which we will photograph on a 35mm film. This way, we can
tell if it is anything in your heart itself, in the muscles, or — as I
suspect — perhaps a blockage or the beginning of a blockage in
one of your coronary arteries. Your cholesterol level is just at
the higher limits of normal, and an arteriogram is something I
feel you should have." Then he waited. And I waited, mulling
over what he'd said. I could see the catheter as it entered the
artery, twisting and turning to enter my heart.

Then I asked him: "Have you done many of these, Richard?"

And with relief, he laughed and said: "I can't recall the
number; there are so many times I've done this."

I had developed a sense of complete trust in his judgment.
"Whatever you and Dr. Kanter feel should be done, I will agree
to."

He made a small note on the chart that he held in his hand,
and then, as he was leaving the room, he said: "I'll stop by later
in the day and take another look at you." We said our good-byes
and I fell asleep again.

In the late afternoon, Richard returned. There were the
usual questions and I gave my usual answers, that I felt fine and
that I was still wondering what I was doing in the hospital. I
asked him: "When you do this arteriogram, suppose you find
that there is nothing wrong?" He didn't answer, but reached for
his stethoscope. I asked again: "Could it be nothing?"

As he put the stethoscope to his ears, he said, quietly, "I
don't think so."

Now it was time for a new language to be learned. The

Tower of Babel could not have been more confusing than the tongues I heard in the next 48 hours.

That evening, I signed the release form so that the catheterization could be performed. As the nurse was about to take the form back, I held onto it for a moment and read the contents slowly. Simply stated, it said that Dr. Landesman was authorized to perform the arteriogram and any other necessary procedures that he felt were required. But the second paragraph of the consent form haunted me. In essence it said that the physician had explained to me the reasons for performing such procedures, the possible alternatives to such procedures, and certain risks and consequences that might be involved in or arise from such procedures, including the following (and underneath was written in Richard Landesman's handwriting):

1. Heart attack.
2. Loss of pulse.

When I returned the form to the nurse, suddenly, again, I felt apprehension and fear about the procedure. And yet I knew within my own thinking that even if it were a simple appendectomy, there is no such thing as a simple procedure and that any procedure that invades the body has certain complications. Quickly, I went through the pluses: My EKG was normal, there were no enzyme changes (meaning, there never had been destruction of heart tissue, at least up to the present moment); I seemed to be in excellent physical condition; I'd never had a heart attack; and I trusted Richard Landesman with my life.

The following morning I am groggy, sleepy; the injection the nurse had given me upon awakening was beginning to take effect, and I seemed to recall being in a twilight state. As my eyes opened, I found myself staring at a television screen. I did not feel the incision or the beginning of the surgical procedure; I felt nothing except some sleepiness. I fought the sleepiness out of curiosity and, interestingly, felt no apprehension. It was almost as if I were watching from the distance a procedure being performed on someone other than myself. On the television screen I could see a pulsating organ, and I knew it was my heart. Suddenly, a tiny filament began to snake its way on-screen, curling into the aorta, the largest artery, which leads

from the heart to supply the entire body with blood; the filament seemed to stay inside each ventricle. I could hear voices
behind me, talking about the pressure of the blood as it was
being pumped through the chambers of my heart. Occasionally
I would hear Richard's voice saying, "That's fine; that's good."
And then the filament began to snake into a coronary artery
and a small amount of dye appeared at the tip of the catheter.
As I watched, it filled the artery to its end. Then it would be
pulled back and go into another coronary artery.

In the last coronary artery, something appeared on that
screen that was different. I watched the dye entering this particular coronary artery. It seemed about the size of a pencil in
diameter, or a little smaller. Suddenly, the dye disappeared.
About a half-inch down the artery it reappeared and filled the
pencil-sized artery. I watched the dye reach to the end of the
various tributaries and then disappear.

It seemed that the entire process of catheterization was performed very quickly, and I cannot remember too much at this
point.

I awoke in my room. Richard stood before me and told me
that I had a marked constriction of the left anterior descending
coronary artery. He also told me that having a problem with
this artery is a very serious matter, since this artery feeds the
left ventricle, which is needed to pump blood up to the aorta
and throughout the body. There is some medicine that I am
acquainted with, and I recall from my days as a medical student
that this blood vessel was often referred to as the "widow's
artery" — the cause of sudden death.

I said nothing to Richard. He explained that this particular
artery showed a marked constriction and that a surgical procedure called a coronary bypass is the recommended method for
alleviating this hazardous constriction. "It is basically simple,"
Richard explained. The operation consists of taking a vein from
the leg and attaching it to the coronary artery above the constriction. The other part of the vein is attached below the constriction, so that the blood supply will not be interrupted by
this damaged vessel which is slowly blocking itself off.

Suddenly, it seemed so elementary, so necessary, so essential.
We talk of two men out in the Midwest, in Milwaukee: Johnson

and Shore. The cardiologist knows them; Don Kanter, my internist, knows them; but I do not. I know Freud and Jung and Harry Stack Sullivan — even my own orientation develops step by step upon these lines — but Johnson and Shore? Who are these mystics of the Midwest that the world seems to venerate? Was that the proper way to describe it? It was certainly the impression I was getting from Richard. Truly, I had become a child again, bewildered gleefully by the hand that's quicker than the eye. But I now agree. Richard calls Dr. Shore; it is agreed. Science marches on; I sweep along, feeling no anxiety or fear, trusting my physician's judgment implicitly. That is right, is it not?

At 11:30 A.M. the next day I leave the hospital and I am told that I am to fly to Milwaukee, to arrive at St. Mary's Hospital on Christmas Day.

It is now December 20th and I am home.

I am now taking Inderal. I have a supply of nitroglycerin tablets to be placed under my tongue if I should feel any further discomfort. I am told to take two aspirins daily (this is to help prevent the blood from clotting excessively). I have five days to wait before we fly to Milwaukee. Carol is concerned, insisting that I rest. I am becoming totally bored with just staying home; I am anxious with this boredom; it is not my nature to do nothing. I want to drive into town; I want to go to my office; I want to do a multitude of things. In essence, I want to feel that I am normal and that nothing is wrong. I know that I cannot fool myself, that there is something terribly wrong, and that it has to be corrected. I have to rest and avoid any kind of stress — to be patient.

My two sons, who have arrived from school, keep me occupied with stories of their experiences with their friends, their classes, and their professors. My dearest friends, Lucille and Ron King, visit almost every evening for approximately a half hour. I want them to stay, but intuitively, they know that it is best not to remain too long. I spend much of the day sleeping, watching television, or reading. I do anything to distract my attention from myself. But the mechanism of denial does not work with me; I cannot simply pretend that a condition does not exist.

The day before I leave for Milwaukee, Lucille and Ron King visit again. This time Ron brings his briefcase. Very frankly and quietly he says that he has reviewed my will, and he asks me to sign the power-of-attorney paper for Carol. I smile at him and mutter, "Just in case, Ron?" He does not know what to say and pretends not to hear my question. I had not realized until that moment that so many of my business affairs were unsettled, that it was necessary for Ron to review all these affairs with Carol.

I could not bring myself to stay and listen to the conversation between Carol and Ron. I did not want to think about the worst possibility. Hoping to avoid forcing my thoughts in this direction, feeling a sudden flood of depression, I almost ran from the room.

I was feeling tired, concerned that because of inactivity my energy was diminishing. I went to bed while Carol and Ron reviewed the necessary matters that a client and an attorney discuss under these circumstances. Gratefully, I slept deeply.

When I awake it is 10:00 P.M. I go downstairs; my sons and wife are talking quietly. With a silly grin, I say, "Merry Christmas, everybody! Let's open the packages tonight." We spend the remainder of the evening opening all the gifts. The joyful distraction is most appreciated, and by midnight I am once again asleep.

Two

The Artery That Can Kill

Carol and I arrive just before noon at St. Mary's Hospital in Milwaukee. The weather in Milwaukee is cold, bitterly cold, and snow lies all around. Cold and snow are elements not exactly beneficial to cardiac patients. We are expected. Carol gives the canister that contains the 35-mm film of my catheterization to the receptionist, who states that it will be sent to Dr. Shore's office in the hospital.

Science marches on. There is the usual routine of hospital admissions. Laboratory work, x-rays, interviews, insurance forms, Blue Cross, on and on. Knowing full well that these questions must be answered, I cannot help but indicate a little of my irritation. Where are my gods? Where are my surgeons? I realize that it is Christmas Day. They, too, have families.

Carol tries to amuse me. We play Scrabble, and we talk. I find myself reassuring her; she seemed a delicate flower, slowly wilting. By 9:30 P.M., I send her home, to a local inn. It is perhaps the third time we have slept apart in our entire marriage. Is this all a nightmare? Where is faith, hope, and dignity for me? What sort of man is this Dr. Shore? I only know what I have been told. Reputations are for others. Immediacy and the present human contact are my needs and I grow very weary. Christmas Day ends, but I continue. Reality goes on. The loneliness of being in that hospital room is the most painful experience; pain is the loneliest experience, one that cannot be shared. I would wish neither pain nor loneliness on any human soul. I took a Dalmane for sleep: sweet dreams of my children.

The following day I awoke early at St. Mary's Hospital — just the place where a nice Jewish psychiatrist should find himself! Carol arrived early and tried to divert my mind and my attention from what I knew I had to go through. At the same time, I was still furious that I had not been visited by an intern, a resident, a cardiologist, or this Dr. Shore who was going to split me in half and take a look at my coronary arteries.

The door opened. It was about three in the afternoon, and in Milwaukee at three in the afternoon in late December it begins to get rather dark. In walked Dr. Richard Shore, accompanied by a nurse. I found out later that she is his particular liaison nurse; she takes care of his patients and is actually a go-between for the patient and the physician. If there are any complaints, or if there is anything to be followed up, it is her job to follow the orders and the suggestions that Dr. Shore would lay out for the patients. She is the essence of tact.

Seeing Dr. Shore, I remember thinking to myself how strange it is that one has preconceived ideas of what other people will look like, but I had no more right to imagine what Richard Shore would look like than he had to imagine what I would look like. He stood there, very pleasant — attractive, as a matter of fact — and clean shaven. As I sat in bed looking up at him, I saw few wrinkles on his face. He looked young, and yet I knew, or was told, that he was in his middle forties, but I'm not too sure if that was just plain gossip or guesses handed to me by the nurses.

My first impulse was to say to him, "Where the hell have you been! I've been sitting here over 24 hours waiting to see somebody and you finally come in. I don't think that's very nice of you." But I didn't say that. I wouldn't say that. I couldn't say that. Instead, I said, "I trust you had a pleasant Christmas."

Now can you imagine such a shmucky thing to say, considering the anger that I felt those 24 hours? Certainly, I was not going to insult the man who was going to take a knife to me, the man whose fingers and hands and brains I was going to rely upon, the man whom I hoped God had touched in a very special way. And at that particular moment we have thoughts that fly across our minds with great rapidity, and yet they have to pass through a memory track somewhere in one's brain. I imagined Richard Shore as the Adam painted by Michaelangelo, his hands in surgical gloves, a forefinger extended as God reaches out to touch him and give him this tremendous talent and very special ability so that he can do what he is going to do for me — hopefully give me another chance, and hopefully, too, hundreds of other patients another chance.

I am not totally selfish — not really — but at that moment I was selfish enough to think only of me, not of the hundreds of other patients whom I knew those golden fingers would help.

He was very pleasant. He said he had a very nice Christmas and asked whether I was being taken care of, whether all the x-rays and blood tests had been done, and whether I was annoyed by all the laboratory work that I had to go through. How, I said to myself, can I be angry at this man who is asking me if everything is all right and if the staff is treating me properly?

"The staff is quite marvelous," I said, and meant it sincerely. "I cannot pick any one particular nurse or technician who is better than any other. Each is uniquely good, capable, and very much aware of what they have to do and do it."

I was in my pajamas and bathrobe. He took a stethoscope from his pocket, asked me to open my bathrobe and pajama top, and listened to my chest and back to check if my lungs were clear. I knew what he was doing. As a physician I knew that he was checking for any particular pathology in a heartbeat or any sound that did not belong there, and he was checking my lungs to see that they were not filling with fluid. After he finished he checked my ankles to see whether they were swollen and I could see him gently apply pressure to my shinbone to see whether there was any fluid. I knew everything he was doing, and he knew I knew it too. We spoke just a little while — not very long — about the origin of my symptoms. I told him I had no pain, and I told him exactly what had happened. He listened with the kind of intensity that I hope I have when listening to my own patients. I was very proud to be a colleague of his and proud to have him as my physician.

After he completed the examination he asked, "Did you bring the films?" I told him that I had given the receptionist the film of the angiogram that had been done in Stamford Hospital.

He turned to the nurse who had come with him and asked, "Have you seen the films, Kathy?"

She answered, "No, Doctor, but I do know they are in the screening room."

"Fine," he replied, and, turning to me, he asked whether I would like to go with him to look at the films. I jumped out of bed, with a grateful smile, so pleased that he was willing to treat me as an equal and not as a lay patient who would not understand. He was willing to share with me and perhaps to encourage my asking questions, to alleviate anxiety on my part.

Just as I was about to swing out of bed, he noticed my pipe and tobacco pouch lying on the bedside stand. (I've always felt pipe smoking to be far superior to cigarette smoking, and I found it relaxing and rather enjoyed the taste and smell of good pipe tobacco, as opposed to what I thought of as the stench of cigarettes.) He pointed to the pipe on the bedside table. "Is this yours?" he asked.

"Yes," I answered.

"Do you blow soap bubbles with it?"

I looked up at him and said, "I don't think I will be using it for blowing soap bubbles."

"Well, in that case," he said, taking the pipe and dropping it into the wastepaper basket, "it is a rather foolish thing for a physician, isn't it?"

I agreed, as I heard the pipe hit the bottom of the wastepaper basket.

"And besides," he continued, "smoking is not permitted, of course. If I knew you were smoking, I don't think I would want to operate upon you."

"Oh, I have not smoked," I said, protesting weakly. I knew full well that he was aware I was lying, but it set the tone of an understanding between us that the pipe in that wastebasket had seen its last day. As be began to move toward the door he picked up the tobacco pouch, which had very little tobacco left in it, and threw it into the wastepaper basket also. "You won't need this soap powder, either," he said and opened the door to the room.

Carol and I accompanied him and Kathy to the screening room. In silence we walked down the hall, into the elevator. I watched him push a button. The elevator went down to some floor. We all got out. He led the way, Kathy beside him, down a long corridor and we stopped in front of a door labelled "Video-screen." In the room was a wall of canisters containing films of thousands of patients; I became apprehensive, wondering whether my films were there, and then Kathy picked them up. They were on top of the video-screening machine. She opened the canister that had my name on it and adjusted the reel. Then Dr. Shore ran the film through quickly by hand; I watched the screen with him. Neither of us said a word. This was the first time I had seen them; I was completely oblivious even to Carol at that moment, although I'm sure *she* watched them rather anxiously. He rewound the film and we saw everything go backward; then he ran it forward again, and again he rewound it backward. The third time he ran it very slowly, and this time he spoke.

He said, "Here, you can see, Dr. Waxberg, the catheter coming into the aorta and going into the left anterior descending coronary artery. Do you see that?" The film stopped, and I could see the tip of the catheter. The memory of this picture when taken at Stamford Hospital was vague.

Then he said, "Now, as I turn it, watch the way the dye enters that particular left anterior descending coronary artery." And he turned the film slowly by hand and I could see the dye come out of the tip of the catheter and fill the artery. The artery seemed about the thickness of an ordinary pencil. Suddenly the artery came to a point; it looked like a thread approximately an inch in length or it seemed that way to me — it may have been a quarter of an inch; it may have been a half inch; it may have been a foot — I do not know, I cannot recall. It seemed to go on forever. How big is a coronary artery? But there it was. The

coronary artery was the size of a pencil, and suddenly it narrowed down to a thread. The dye filled the coronary artery, and
then one couldn't see it go through the part that was so narrow.
The artery opened up again to the size of a pencil behind the
thread, and the dye went through the thread, into the remainder
of that particular artery that seemed to be the normal size.

I became terrified. That artery was so clogged! Wasn't it
amazing that I had no symptoms? Wasn't it amazing that the
artery hadn't closed entirely by now? Wasn't it amazing that I
was still alive? Wasn't it amazing that I was watching this? And
wasn't it amazing that Dr. Shore was so nonchalant about this?

Again he pointed to the thread and said, "I guess we're
going to have to do a bypass. Perhaps we can use your internal
mammary artery and bring it down to this point." He pointed
to an area past the thread to show me he was going to bypass
that area where the artery was slowly choking itself off. Pro-
fessionally, with a very calm, soft voice, he told me this. "Looks
like the other arteries seem to be pretty good. I can't see anything to be concerned about, but when we get inside, if I should
see anything else that requires a little adjusting and fixing — why,
I trust that you will permit me to do so."

I remained speechless, because I kept staring at the left
anterior descending coronary artery up on that screen. In the
middle of that artery, that thread was choked with all sorts of
plaques and cholesterol deposits and clots: all sorts of horrible pathology I remembered hearing about as a medical student. I wondered how in the world I was breathing and still
living. Isn't it fantastically fortunate that I'm still alive? Had I
not had that unfamiliar "indigestion" that particular evening,
I would not have known that this was inside me. One day I
simply would not wake up.

"I am wondering," I said aloud to Dr. Shore, "Why the
internal mammary artery? It seems such a strange artery, running along the ribcage, one on each side of the sternum. Why
this particular artery?"

"I use it," he explained, "as the bypass graft of *choice* with
left anterior descending coronary disease, such as you see on the
screen." He sensed that this was not a sufficient explanation for
me and continued: "Would you like statistics, Doctor?"

I answered, smiling, "Yes I would, Doctor." I appreciated his concern that I understand everything that he was going to do. It was important to me and also important for him to explain it so that both of us could have a complete understanding. I knew this would increase my trust in him and confidence in the surgery that I was to undergo.

"Well," he began, "perhaps it would be best to say that the internal mammary artery has a much lower chance of closure or clogging after surgery than a saphenous vein from your leg. The differences in percentages are perhaps small, but nevertheless the percentages are on the side of the internal mammary artery, and this is why we use it. Another reason is that the blood flow in the mammary grafted artery increases as the need occurs because it is an artery and as such is naturally suited to adapt to arterial flow. The vein grafts, on the other hand, tend to thicken at times and narrow. Although this may take many years, we found a percentage of success with the mammary artery in this hospital. I must also tell you, Joe," he said, his voice more friendly, but still professional, "that mammary artery grafts do produce some chest-wall pain and a slightly higher incidence of increased time for healing." I was pleased at his honesty in this small lecture he was giving me.

"In the last ten years of using the mammary artery," he continued, "we have not documented a single failure, but with the saphenous vein, on the other hand, we can see occasionally, in two or three percent of the patients, deterioration over a year. Another factor, for some reason that we do not quite understand, is that the mammary artery seems to be somewhat immune to plaque and cholesterol deposits. Perhaps because it is an artery that feeds the breasts, which are necessary for the reproduction and continuation of our species, mother nature has endowed this particular artery in this manner."

"You say that I will need only this one bypass," I said.

"As far as I can see from these films," he answered. "But, again, once I have an opportunity to examine all the coronary arteries, I will be able to see whether there is any early development of sclerosis or blocking. When you sign the permission for the surgery, you will notice that it stipulates that in the event I do find some other artery that requires a bypass, it will be done. So far I see only this one, but after surgery, if you find that I have done more, I don't want you to be surprised or even apprehensive about it. On other bypasses, if they are needed, I will use the saphenous vein."

Again, I saw one of my fleeting mental images. Once again, I saw Michaelangelo's Adam and God about to make contact (but, of course, it is Dr. Shore again and not Adam), and this time there is dialogue added. God is saying to Dr. Shore, "I command you to take care of my boy, Joe, down there, and you can do it because he is not finished with the work that he has to do on earth."

Can you imagine the audacity of me in a video screening room having this picture flashing through my mind with the speed of light? I thanked Dr. Shore for his interpretation and for his patience. "Do you mind if I ask you one more question?"

He responded, as patiently as ever, "If I can answer, I certainly will try."

I asked him, "Is there another way? Does there exist another way to treat this condition?"

I remember watching Carol out of the corner of my eye, and I could imagine her thoughts: Where do you get the audacity to ask such a question of this man? Meanwhile, I am looking at Dr. Shore, waiting for his reply. He smiled at me, and I remember saying to myself, "He has such nice white teeth, because he doesn't smoke."

"Well," he said, "I suppose we could use Drano!"

Now there is very little that you can say after you have made an idiot of yourself. I thanked him for his patience and kindness and for taking the time to explain everything to me and to Carol. Turning to leave the video screening room, Kathy opened the door and said, "Just walk down to the elevator; you'll find it to your right. Go up to the fifth floor and you'll find your way back to your room."

Carol and I walked down the hall, saying nothing to each other. Getting into the elevator, we still said nothing to each other; getting off the elevator, still nothing. We got off on the fifth floor and walked toward the room in silence. I took off my bathrobe and got into bed. Then Carol said, "You know, sometimes, Joe, you have an amazing manner. I think it would

be most irritating coming from any other human being, but
when it comes from your mouth, nobody seems to be offended.
Is this something special that you have taught yourself or
developed?" I looked at her in amazement and replied, "That's
one of my charms."

A few moments later the nurse brought in my dinner tray. I
begged Carol to share my dinner; I had very little appetite and
ate little. I preferred to share it with Carol so she wouldn't have
to go downstairs to the cafeteria. I also did not want to have to
get up and walk around, because that thread of the coronary
artery was embossed on my mind. I was not going to show her
the absolute terror I was feeling.

Medication was brought in. Pills came at me and I simply
took them and swallowed them down. I got rather drowsy. I
realized at this point that this was already my second day at
St. Mary's Hospital, the day after Christmas, and I was going to
be operated on the third day after Christmas. And in my haze I
asked Carol, "What does the third day of Christmas bring?
The first day is the partridge in a pear tree, but what does the
third day bring?" I did not hear her answer, because I dozed
off.

When I opened my eyes it was dark. Through the window I
could see a few street lights, and under the door of the hospital
room I could see the yellow-orange light weakly shining across
the floor. I found myself wide awake, with the most tremendous
erection bulging through my pajamas pants! Psychiatric patients
who had gone through surgery had often told me similar stories.
Now this is the most ludicrous thing to occur, I thought. Why
do I have this erection when I am preparing myself for an experience that I wouldn't wish on my worst enemy. I lay quietly
and placed my hand on this massive piece of flesh and said to
myself, Surely it does contain a bone. It amused me, and for the
first time in what seemed ages I found myself smiling in the
darkness at myself, at the idiocy of the moment and the de-
liciousness of what I felt in my body.

The fantastic, lustful feeling that I was experiencing at
that moment was so pleasurable that I immediately thought of
Carol. I wanted to reach for the phone, dial the number of the
Milwaukee Inn, and talk to her. I wanted to tell her about this

beautiful piece of tissue, tell her how wonderful I felt and how much I loved her and how much I wanted her and how much at that moment I would have loved to make love to her.

But I couldn't do such a thing. That would have been stupid. I got out of bed. Perhaps I need to urinate, I thought; that will make this tumescence pass. I did not have to urinate at all, so I just stood there, contemplating that growth poking out of my pajamas, and amused myself with memories of earlier years.

Scientifically, I knew that the erection was easily explainable. Apparently I had a dream; we know that erections are frequently associated with dreams. We can tell whether a patient is dreaming if he exhibits rapid eye movements, noticeable through his eyelids. Once analytical thinking had begun, all sorts of data and information began to pour into my conscious mind.

For example, one out of five men in the United States will have a heart attack before he reaches the age of sixty. In this country alone, there are forty million patients whose hearts are affected with coronary artery disease or with high blood pressure that can lead to strokes and other difficulties. It seems interesting that I should be thinking of the small amount of money that perhaps the insurance company would reimburse me compared to the forty-five billion dollars that are spent annually in this country to treat patients with problems affecting their heart. Men generally are susceptible to heart disease; women after menopause exhibit similar susceptibility. Prior to menopause, estrogen prevents the excessive formation of cholesterol deposits in women; men, of course, never have the protection of the female hormones. Statistics — I recalled Dr. Shore asked whether I wanted them. Yes I did. And I added more to the ones he gave me. I knew for example, that men in the United States, Great Britain, Canada, and Finland rank highest in the rate of coronary artery disease; the rate is lowest for men in Sweden and Holland. Perhaps they eat more fish and less meat filled with fat. That is for others to work upon.

I could not shake the memory of the film in the video screening room. I could see those red blood cells flowing through the coronary arteries. I hoped they would not clump up and occlude that artery! The red blood cells in one human being laid end to end, would circle the globe four times. An amazing statistic.

I gripped the button tightly to ring for the nurse. My apprehension was growing as these statistics came to mind. I could feel my heart beat; how long could this organ of muscle tissue continue contracting at its rate of hundred thousand beats per day?

I must stop this line of thought, I told myself. I reached for another button, the one that turned on the television set, adjusted the volume, and began to watch an old black and white film, from a year that I do not remember, except that I do recall seeing Barbara Stanwyck. I was bored by the story and thought the acting was overdone. Slowly my eyes closed and I fell asleep.

Three

Getting to Know the Bird Man

There was one person at the hospital who became especially important to me. He was a gentleman about fifty or so, whose job was to teach me to use the "bird." The bird was a respiratory machine that forced oxygen and fluid into one's lungs after surgery, to keep them expanded and moist and to help the healing process and the use of the lungs, which have to be collapsed during surgery in the bypass operation. The bird is a breathing machine that breathes for you. Your lungs do not move in the normal fashion; the heart-lung machine does all the work for you.

I called him the Bird Man. He resembled a large, friendly stork, having a long neck, a long, pointed nose, and a friendly voice that squeaked a little. He got me to use the bird practically every four hours to keep my lungs expanded and the smallest areas in the lungs sprayed with fluid so that they would not become too dry.

I would sit with the mouthpiece tucked between my lips, letting this machine blow the air down deep into my lungs. Then the machine would click off and allow the air to come out of my nose. It would take approximately five seconds for that

machine to fill my lungs and three seconds for the air to be expelled. I would count to myself; meanwhile, the Bird Man
would tell me stories. "Did you know," he said, one time,
"seven years ago I had this operation? I needed to have several
bypasses, which Dr. Shore did. I felt very strongly that it was
my duty to repay the hospital and to help other patients with
the use of this bird machine. I have to be very honest," he confided, "The respiratory therapist who worked with me was not
too efficient and not very pleasant. And I was very anxious
about the use of this machine because I knew it was very essential to me. So I decided to study respiratory therapy at school
and learn how to demonstrate this. Now I devote three days a
week. On the other days I have a little television repair shop
which supports me."

I am always overwhelmed by people who, out of a tremendous sense of gratitude, have a need to repay society or an
organization or an individual through work. There can be no
other way for these people—giving money or simply visiting
and holding hands are not enough. The Bird Man felt that
improvement was needed, so he went to school at night to learn
to become an inhalation therapist. Indeed, he was a remarkable
man. Each time I saw him it was a pleasant respite from the
day. To be very frank, the first few days after surgery are rather
painful. There is so much going on inside your whole chest; it
feels stirred up, as though a half dozen children had been digging
in it as in a sandbox, and they'd left their toys and pails and
shovels just hanging and tipped over, lying on the side in a distressing manner, helter-skelter.

In the beginning it was very difficult for me to learn the
technique of the use of this inhalator. It seemed as though my
chest became a balloon; I just couldn't handle all the air that
was forced down into my lungs, and I would have a fit of
coughing. The Bird Man was very patient, and he explained
little tricks: I shouldn't fight the air going into my lungs, but
just let the machine breathe for me; if I should tense up and become anxious, the muscles of my trachia leading down to my
lungs would tighten and not permit enough air to enter. Every
few hours when he arrived with the machine, I would practice
diligently, and with his assistance I soon became adept at just

relaxing and letting the inhalation machine force the air in and then click off. The air would be expelled, and then the machine would click on and the entire process repeated over and over again. He kept up a steady, pleasant kind of chatter, telling me about his own bypass and how pleased he was with the results. I was extremely grateful to him because nothing is more distressing than to hear about complications and problems with surgery that one is about to undergo. He had nothing but the highest praise for the entire staff — nurses, technicians, and physicians — and nothing but praise for the attention that was meted out to him. I looked forward to his visits, to his kindly voice and to his constant reassurance. I became very adept at the use of the machine.

The Bird Man first appeared on the second day of my hospitalization, December 26. It was necessary that I learn how to use this machine before surgery because it was going to play an extremely important part in my treatment after the operation. Although at first I hesitated and found myself finding all sorts of reasons and excuses not to take this seriously, by the third visit of the Bird Man, using the machine would become an urgent activity on my part. I decided that I could not afford to ignore this very important procedure. I was going to cooperate. I was going to stop acting like an imposed-upon child. I shall always be indebted to the Bird Man for what he taught me and, more important than that, for the way he helped me.

When I had arrived at St. Mary's Hospital it had been Christmas Day, so very little had been done, but things happened very rapidly in the next few days since I was scheduled for surgery on the morning of December 28. Still, I found myself bored with the waiting, anxious, and irritated at being able to do nothing except try to tolerate the passage of time. It was at these moments that I would leave my room and walk around the corridors of the hospital.

The hospital was built so that those patients who were undergoing bypass surgery were grouped in two sections. They were adjacent to each other, yet apart, and they were differently painted. The section I was in was blue and the other was a light green. As I wandered from one section to the other, I began to

meet other patients who were in various stages of the operation.
There were some who were waiting to be operated on, some
who had just returned from the Intensive Care Unit after surgery, and some who were preparing themselves for departure.
I got an impression of the continuous flow handled by the
staff; each patient's work was assigned and followed through
with a dedication that I did not appreciate until it was my turn
to leave.

It was during my wandering that I met three other patients
who all lived near me in Fairfield County, Connecticut. Two of
them lived in Stamford, and one lived in Norwalk. I lived in
New Canaan. It was strange that all of us had different cardiologists, and each of us was different from the others in reference
to his illness.

The first one was Vince, a retired deputy police chief in his
late fifties, short of build, always with a pleasant smile on his
round face. He loved to have company and tell stories about
his police work. He was cheerful, affable, the kind of fellow
that you wouldn't mind having around. He was also sensitive
enough to know when to withdraw or when to stop talking or
to change the subject if he felt it was producing anxiety in
another patient. He worked on a very primitive level, instinc-
tively reacting to other people's facial reactions and tone of
voice. Vince was an extremely empathic individual and did not
know or even attempt to analyze why or how he had developed
this particular capability. All he knew was that he needed bypasses for his angina.

Vince introduced me to the second patient, Bill, a salesman.
He was short and very thin, with a history of one heart attack
and one very mild stroke that had left certain areas of the right
side of his face sort of numbed but had not affected the muscles;
you couldn't tell that he had had a stroke that involved deep
muscle paralysis. It was basically a sensory paralysis — a feeling
of numbness. Like Vince, he had a long history of angina, and
the pain was rather debilitating for him. He also had a problem
with his aorta. The aorta is the largest artery in the body. It
comes off the heart and goes down the center of the body,
lying against the spinal cord, and when it gets to the pelvis it
splits into two arteries, each going to a leg. At the level of the

split, his aorta had developed some sort of blockage, but they could not operate on him until they had taken care of the problems with his coronary arteries. Bill was a pleasant fellow, but somewhat withdrawn — not because he didn't like to talk and horse around, but because his mind was on himself; it was very difficult to distract his attention. No matter what we would be talking about, his eyes would cloud over, and he would pull inside himself. You could imagine his brain forming little tracks to some area of his mind instead of to his ears. Occasionally, when Vince asked him a question, Bill would have to apologize because his mind had been distracted. Vince had an amazing facility for accepting Bill's self-absorption — he would almost apologize for intruding into Bill's thoughts.

The third friend I met, Tony, a building contractor, was the youngest of us all, in his forties. We never discussed age, except in terms of mine, so that if I would say I was fifty-five, Vince would say, "Well, I'm older than that"; Bill would say, "I'm just a bit younger than that"; and Tony would say, "Jesus, I'm not even fifty." This interchange set the tone for the four of us. Tony was a heavy-set fellow, very overweight, and he smoked too much. He had tremendous amounts of angina, constantly. We all admitted to this throughout the days we spent together. We ranked ourselves according to the amount of angina we suffered. Bill and Tony had equal amounts.

Frequently, after the mornings, which were usually occupied with various tests, we would have a few hours when we would get together in somebody's room or occasionally in a little alcove off the hallway, just to talk.

They all knew I was a physician, and in the beginning there was a certain kind of reticence in talking because they had been told I was a psychiatrist. But as time progressed — I measured time in those days in minutes, perhaps in hours — it became apparent to them that I was not acting in the role of a therapist. I was one of them; my anxieties were the same as theirs. I could answer a bit of some of their questions, and if there were questions on matters about which I had no knowledge, when one of the cardiologists appeared, all of us wanted answers. It pleased them to see that I was as ignorant of cardiac surgery as they were.

I found myself developing very specific reactions to my three friends. With Vince, I was a very close friend. There was discussion, of course, (about his family, my family, and our respective children), but there were also personal feelings between us. There was also a complete exchange of philosophical thought, and together we attempted to analyze what the metaphor of the experience meant to each of us.

Bill was more introspective and more educated than the other two. He had gone through the most physical difficulty, and he was much more anxious than the rest of us. He tried to convince us that his angina was under control, but I could not help noticing his taking nitroglycerin tablets. His concern, as I pointed out, was with himself, but when the two of us were alone he would not withdraw as much as he would when all four of us met. Perhaps he was more open with me because of the many hours we spent alone, talking about the things that had happened to him, and because I identified with more than just his heart problems. When there was a third or fourth member of the quartet on the floor, he withdrew, preventing our continuing any discussion we had already started. I could feel that he was offended at the intrusion of the others, and I must confess too that there were times when I had a similar feeling if we were deep into some particular subject.

Now Tony, whom we referred to as the "baby," was very shy, withdrawn, easily manipulated by others around him. I found myself in a protective role; I am not sure whether I chose it for him or for myself. There were other patients on the floor who would go into his room during the times he should have been resting. They would keep him awake, or insist that he go with them to an area of the floor where one was permitted to smoke. (Vince and I did not smoke; Bill did occasionally, but not with Tony's intensity.) Once, after Tony had gone through a rather strenuous examination and should have been exhausted, I found another patient in the room sprawled out on Tony's bed while Tony sat in an uncomfortable chair. In my role as protector, I became angry and asked the visitor to leave, pointing out that Tony needed bed rest and that if the patient wanted to rest in bed he should go to his own room. The patient looked at Tony for some response, and slowly got out of bed, and left the room. When I scolded Tony for not telling him to leave, Tony said, "I couldn't hurt his feelings." Tony got into his bed and even as I was opening the door to leave, I could see his eyes were closed and he was half-way into sleep.

Of course, with Tony one never discussed the upcoming surgery or the reasons for the operation. He never asked about it. He knew it was something that had to be done; unless it was performed, the chances were that he would die young. He had an older brother who underwent a bypass operation, so he was not totally ignorant of what was in store.

I felt a sense of responsibility for my three friends, a responsibility *to* them: to encourage them to eat properly, to stay away from smoking, to cooperate in the testing, to get the rest that was required, to make certain that the medications were taken, no matter how horrible they tasted. This was my quartet.

And this is the way we all arrived in surgery. I went first, followed that afternoon by Vincent; the following day Tony was scheduled. Bill did not know when he was going to be operated on; the surgeons told him they were not even sure that they could operate on him. During the testing he had showed carotid artery involvement (the carotid artery supplies the brain with the necessary blood supply); in addition, his iliac arteries, which supplied both legs, were blocked and he felt a certain numbness and pain in his calf muscles if he walked any distance. It wasn't until I had returned from the ICU and was back in my own room that I was told he had been taken down to surgery on an emergency basis one evening because several coronary arteries had been closing off dangerously. The surgeons had been very concerned that this was extremely dangerous to his heart muscle; they had had to work fast and, fortunately, Bill had come through all right.

I did not know in those days, while we patients talked and developed friendships, that a seed was being planted in my mind. When the seed sprouted (providing I survived surgery), like the Bird Man, I was going to devote time talking to other bypass patients. At that time it was premature to formulate ideas that were only beginning to grow, but later there was a genuine flowering: First, we formed a small group; as the years progressed, we became a fairly large group of bypass patients (and their wives) who helped others during the difficult recovery stages. But at that moment the seed had been planted and I simply let Mother Nature cultivate the seed without my participation.

There was one other procedure that all patients had to go through prior to surgery, and that was to have an intravenous injection of a nuclear medication that would spread throughout the body. The doctors were interested in how this medication would appear on a machine that showed, through a tremendous computerized mechanism, the picture of the heart muscles. I lay on the table with the huge radiation counter clicking away over my chest. On the wall to my right there was a huge screen with multiple dots of various colors; its meaning escaped me entirely (nuclear medicine is a new specialty). The entire process took approximately 20 minutes. As I was taken off the table and placed in the wheel chair, I asked the nurse to stop at the office of the chief of nuclear medicine. In a small office whose walls were lined with a multitude of diplomas and awards, I saw for the first time the diploma awarded to him as a specialist in nuclear medicine. Once I introduced myself as a colleague he was eager to explain his work. He could not tell me about the results of the test on me, of course, since it was still going through the computer at that time, but he could speak in general terms. He explained that each of the red, yellow, green, and blue dots that I'd seen on the screen indicated the health of the muscle tissue, the valves, the arteries and the pericardium, the lining that surrounds the heart itself. The pericardium is sometimes involved in scarring; when a patient has had a heart attack in which a vessel has been blocked off, the muscle tissues that were supplied by this blocked artery ultimately die and become scar tissue. Because scar tissue does not absorb the nuclear medication, it is seen as a black area in the midst of those colored dots. He could pretty well pinpoint the area of the heart that was involved. He showed me various photographs of different hearts he had worked on; attached to each photograph was the surgeon's report corroborating the evidence that had initially been discovered through nuclear medicine. It was still a very new technique at the time, and he spoke in enthusiastic terms about the use of this machine as a diagnostic tool for future cardiac patients. This included not only those who would have to undergo surgery, but those patients who could be treated medically.

I stared at him as he spoke enthusiastically, regretting my own inability (not being more diligent in physics) to see and understand, through his explanations, how important this diagnostic tool was, and how important it would become in the future. I was returned to my room just in time for another visit from my good friend, the Bird Man.

Four

The Day Before Surgery

On December 27, the day before surgery, I awoke early. I went to the window, peering over the flat Milwaukee scene. It was 6:30 in the morning. I watched the shadows of the buildings get shorter as the sun rose in the sky. In the distance, a highway was filled with morning traffic. Most of the cars still had their lights on, and I saw an endless stream coming down the highway. I caught myself comparing them to red corpuscles coursing through coronary arteries.

I felt very jittery and tense. I did not understand the apprehension I was feeling; it was a new experience for me. In anticipation of the unknown, I found myself wondering about tomorrow, not in terms of the surgery, but in terms of life: Would I survive? Hundreds of thousands of operations are successful, I kept reassuring myself, but I could not seem to shake the doubts that I felt—not so much in the capability of Dr. Shore and his surgical team, but in my own body, in my own physical capacities to deal with this bypass.

The cars poured down the highway; I felt pleasure in seeing that there was no traffic jam, because the flow of traffic symbolized the blood traveling down that coronary artery within

my chest. There was a traffic jam inside me; I visualized the
corpuscles as they approached the blockage as a four-lane highway narrowing down to a single lane. I turned from the window,
unable to cope with the image, and returned to bed.

Now I found my thoughts were about Carol. What if? I
asked myself, and left it hanging. What would happen to Carol
if I did not come through this operation? Rewording the question, What would happen to my wife if I were to die? Let us re-
word it for a third time: Could I do anything? Could I prepare
her? Should I write a little note? What do I do? But it comes
back to the original question: What will happen to my wife if
I die?

I had heard over the years, from other physicians, from
patients, and from friends, several answers to that question.
Now perhaps they were never to be taken seriously, but again
perhaps they were. One example would run like this: "Listen,
the day I die, my wife had better find herself a rich old geezer
who will be able to take care of her the way I've been taking
care of her." Or it might be said another way: "I pity the guy
that my wife grabs onto." The wife becomes a villain, a witch. A
second type of response goes like this: "She certainly has
enough insurance. The business would pay her quite well, rather
handsomely. There will be nothing that she could really want,
so I suspect she'll find herself some young man to keep her
happy." That too seemed the sort of answer one hears from an
unhappy man. The only thing such a man is interested in is that
he has left his wife rich; since the only need that she could
ever conceivably have is for some fantastic sexual expression
that she would have to purchase with the deceased husband's
money. That kind of answer belonged where the first kind of
answer belonged: Nowhere.

There was a third kind of response: "I suppose that that is a
question that my wife would have to resolve for herself." That
answer was certainly better than the others: At least such a
man would be admitting that his wife had the ability and the
intelligence to find some sort of resolution to the problem. But
I did not agree with that kind of answer either. This man was
running away from the problem; he avoided saying what *he*
felt, what *he* hoped. That is the kind of thought that was in-

vading my mind—simply running round and round, without
beginning, without end.

No, I was not going to ponder about a relationship that
has existed for twenty-odd years. One knows that when a couple
has lived and *loved* for more than twenty years, their relationship is unique. It is not made of sticks or a bit of masonry; no,
it is truly bonded, cemented, better than anything held with
any epoxy ever invented. Moments of anger at each other, disappointment with each other, irritation with each other—these
all contribute to the cement that binds two people together
from the very beginning. If it only took an argument or a disagreement to fracture and fragment a relationship, then that
marriage never was of any value or significance. I felt that what
I had was valuable, significant, cemented, bonded, impermeable,
that nothing could tear it asunder—except for death.

These were the thoughts that were occupying my mind. I
was worried and concerned—although not really overly concerned—that I would not live. I still wanted to have the prerog-
ative and option to allow my mind certain thoughts and actions.
I would feel better prepared to talk about and cope with it if
the gears shifted.

I wanted my wife to marry again if it came to that. She is
not a full person, a total personality, alone. She requires another
human being to rebound thoughts, feelings, and experiences.
She needs another human being to share, to talk with. It would
be necessary, I felt, that my wife marry again. I thought this
with no jealousy, no envy, out of concern for her happiness and
her contentment. She and I had had good years, but she had her
life to carry on, and it would not be fair for her to continue
alone. The relationship with our sons or with other relatives
continues, of course, regardless of what happens to the marriage. No, I told myself, she needed a companion. I had no
answers to how she would find one, and I was not going to let
myself be preoccupied with the thought that she might meet
someone who was not going to appreciate her or who would
take advantage of her kindness and generosity. I was not going
to look at the negative aspects of a new relationship. These
things, true, could happen, but my thought was that it was
important for her to know from me that I would want her to

remarry. I would have been more at rest with myself, knowing that she was still content and alive, vivacious and full of fire until her moment came, many years hence. I possessed none of the negative aspects of men who would look for how much money the widow had, or any of the thousands of clichés that do not bear repeating at this stage. I was concerned and I knew that I had to tell her what I felt. How to do this I had not yet resolved.

My thoughts were interrupted by the appearance of breakfast: a bowl of grits on a tray. "Yuch!" As I was eating around the bowl of "yuch," Carol arrived.

"Grits," she said, "my favorite food." I watched in distaste as she finished her favorite food.

"How revolting," I said.

"Better than slimy oysters," she countered as she began to straighten my pillow. As she puttered around me, she asked, "Why don't we go down to the gift shop? I think it would be nice if we bought a few small gifts for all these wonderful nurses and attendants who have been so helpful." I agreed readily, eager to leave the confines of my room. To do so it was required that I be placed in a wheelchair.

In the gift shop we bought about a dozen items for the various nurses and technicians. As I passed the newsstand, I noticed a copy of the *Wall Street Journal*. What made me pick it up was the lead article. It dealt with a coronary bypass report put out by a Veteran's Administration Hospital. It was a devastating article, but I will not go into the details because they have been proven erroneous since then. I read it with great objectivity. As Carol was shopping, I sat in the wheelchair reading, when Dr. Shore came by. We exchanged a few words and I handed him the *Journal.*

He said that he had read the original article in the *New England Journal of Medicine*, but not to take the contents too seriously. Besides, he said, this was not a VA hospital. He turned and said good-bye, and left without my having a chance to question him about the report. His dismissal of the article reassured me. Indeed, I was not in a VA Hospital, and the Shore and Johnson team, which had worked together for many years, had better results than those of the VA; therefore, I concluded that Shore's team was superior in technique and approach in dealing with this problem. I made no mention of the report to Carol. I simply folded the paper in my lap, and wheeled myself over to the perfume counter where she was picking out several bottles for the nurses. When all the purchases were completed and gift-wrapped, we returned to my room.

"You know," I said to her as I climbed into bed, "I thought about you last night. I was thinking about you, the boys, and what would happen to all of you if something drastic happened to me." Her eyes narrowed, and I could sense that this was a topic she preferred not to discuss. I told her about my thoughts: that if I didn't survive the operation, I wanted her to continue her life with another partner.

Suddenly she became angry. "Now, this pessimism must stop," she said. "I will not even continue this dialogue with you."

"But, it is a fact," I replied. "It's something we must talk about."

The silence between us lasted too long. Finally, she said, "I didn't sleep too well last night, and I don't think I will sleep too well tonight, because I too have had these thoughts. I don't know what I would do. I don't want to think about it. Let's please not talk about this any more. You are going to be fine. I love you, and my love will carry you through."

"You are an amazing pragmatist to think your love will make everything well."

"Hasn't it always?" she replied, and I laughed and I admitted to her that it had. We dropped the subject and began to walk around the hallway leaving the small gifts that we had purchased for the various nurses and attendants.

The Bird Man arrived, and we returned to the room. I practiced once again with the respiratory inhalator and was complimented on learning so quickly. I thanked him again for his patience and he left, leaving Carol alone with me but not for too long, because a nurse on duty came in to thank us for our gift. She brought a wrapped bar of soap and instructed me to take a shower now using this soap, and to take another shower using the same soap at six in the evening. It was a large cake of brown soap that seemed to contain pumice and had what appeared to be an iodine base. When I returned from the shower, my skin glowed with an orange tinge. Carol helped dry me.

After I got into my pajamas, Vinnie and his wife Eleanor arrived, and we just sat around talking. Then Vinnie was called to go downstairs to have the nuclear scan to determine whether there was any damage to his heart muscle.

The door opened again and this time Kathy, Dr. Shore's liaison nurse arrived. She asked the usual questions: how did I feel? were there any matters not being cared for? I assured her that everything was going well. She explained that later on in the day I was going to be visited by the anesthesiologist. She regretted that Dr. Shore would not be able to see me today, because he had a rather full surgical schedule. She noticed the orange hue to my skin and reminded me again, as the nurse had previously, to repeat the shower around 6:00 that night. Just as she was ready to leave, she turned once again and said, "I wonder if it would be all right for a senior medical student to do a routine physical? It is part of their education, and as a physician you will understand the importance for these students to learn."

"No objection," I replied. "When will he be around?" She admitted that she did not know, but she did know that he was scheduled to see me sometime that day.

Kathy turned to Carol. "I know tomorrow will be difficult for you. I understand you're staying at the Inn." She opened a small notebook and asked, "What room are you in?"

Carol answered and Kathy made a note of it. "I'll call you about every two hours to let you know how everything is progressing, and when the doctor is taken to the ICU you can visit him."

"Thanks so much, Kathy," Carol said. "I appreciate it. I hesitated to ask — you know, special treatment — acting like a doctor's wife."

Kathy laughed. "Not really. All wives are called. No special treatment. That's my job. Dr. Shore began this years ago."

After she left, I said, "Let's go for a ride."

It seemed the day was moving extremely fast; the sun was setting in the early afternoon in Milwaukee, and I knew that by four o'clock that darkness would deepen.

Now alone, the morning jitteriness returned. I hesitated to get out of bed, suddenly very fearful of exerting myself or doing anything except staying flat and immobile. The room was now totally dark except for some street lights that I could see through the window. I must have dozed off, but probably not for very long, because through the haze of my sleepiness I heard a voice asking whether I was awake. Outlined against the doorway was a young man carrying a medical bag, and I assumed he was the medical student. I turned the light on above the bed and he introduced himself and informed me that he came to do a physical on me. He was a senior medical student and he took an extremely accurate and careful history; his examination was meticulously done, system by system. When he finished, he thanked me for my time and hoped it did not inconvenience me too much. I assured him, it did not. "I understand you teach," he said.

"Yes," I replied.

"Did I pass?" he asked jokingly.

"With flying colors," I replied. We spoke a bit about his school and the fact that he was interested in pediatrics. As we spoke, he put all his tools back into his shiny new bag. We said good-bye and he left the room. It was now time for me to have dinner, which consisted of some soup and Jell-o. I wasn't hungry, but I finished it, and now it was time for my second shower with that brown soap. Then I returned to bed. A soft knock was heard on my door, and in walked the anesthesiologist. He was a huge man, and he towered above me as we spoke. He had a Scottish accent. He inquired as to all my allergies, and made notes on the chart that he held before him. As he spoke, he inquired whether I had abnormal reactions to any of the medications I had taken while at Stamford Hospital. I told him I hadn't.

"At about 5:30 in the morning you'll be coming down to surgery and I'll see you then." I watched as his huge body walked to the door. I wondered whether his head would hit the top of the doorframe, but he just cleared it. Smiling, I turned the light out again; turned on the television set to distract my attention, and watched a film.

It was almost 9:00 now, and a nurse walked into the room carrying a syringe on a tray and a white hospital gown. "If you could change into this gown now," she said, "and leave your pajamas in the closet, I'll be back." I did as she instructed, and in a few minutes she had returned, saw that everything was in order, and gave me a shot in the arm. I hardly felt it, and complimented her for her skill.

She thanked me graciously, and with a sort of a twinkle in her eye, said "When you do thousands you do get good at it. Is there anything else you need?"

I told her, "Not that I know of, except, perhaps a new heart."

She laughed and said, "You'll have that by tomorrow." When she left I put the television set back on, trying to distract my attention, my thoughts, and my anxieties.

As I watched the film, I noticed my eyes beginning to flicker and I realized I was fighting sleep. I shut off the television set, punched the pillow a few times, turned on my side, and fell asleep.

Five

The Simplicity of Bypass Surgery

The room was enormous — not just huge, but enormous! Everything was bathed in a soft orange light; the color did not distress the pupils, though, or cause you to blink or to try to keep your eyes closed. It simply was a color that illuminated everything that you wanted to see. The room seemed as enormous as the Roman Colosseum, even the Astro-Dome, and I lay at the exact center of this room. I could see figures, nurses with crimped bandannas walking from one side of the room to another. I could see male nurses wearing short hats, like those you see in a bakery, their sideburns giving them away. Watching the seemingly endless activity around me, it seemed that each of the halves of my brain could recognize the distinctiveness of the other hemisphere with its own method of thinking and responding. One part seemed to say, "Your genitals are being washed," and the other would seem to answer, "Of course." I had to be shaved from neck to toe. Everything seemed logical — even obvious. A nurse was shaving my pubic region; I felt no personal involvement in the act and had no sense of embarrassment, no feeling that a woman should not be doing this to me. I felt detached, was able to place part of my brain in a corner of the room, and watch the process with complete scientific objectivity about all that was going on. It seemed throughout this time, until I fell into complete unconsciousness, that I was totally aware, capable of understanding the purpose of everything that was being done.

A male nurse appeared. "I am now going to insert a Foley catheter," he said. His voice was even, emotionless, without the modulation I usually associate with voice patterns but the experience was not dream-like by any means: I could hear the voice and I could see the catheter go in, could feel the beginning of it enter into the urethra of my penis. I grunted—not because it hurt, but because of some memory that came bubbling up. I am apprehensive about Foley catheters. When I was a medical student, I had to insert one and I did not do a good job of it. The patient had an enlarged prostate, and I was quite certain I had caused him a great deal of pain. Words floated in this enormous Colosseum, bathed in orange light; all the doctors, nurses, technicians, and assistant technicians, whoever seemed to be within the confines of this huge operating room, indicated or gave me a signal that they knew how I felt and were sympathetic to my feelings. "You do not have an enlarged prostate," I heard myself thinking. "It will not hurt you; they catheterize many patients during any week." It reassured me to feel that each of these contributors knew exactly what he was doing. I could feel the tip of the catheter enter my urethra; it slid gently down the length of my penis. Then I could feel it no more; it was in place. I heard the nurse say, "It's fine now. The urine is coming out. We're in excellent position." The anxieties became diffused by the anesthesia and additional pain-killing drugs. This twilight state did the one thing for me that I could not have done for myself: the memory of that medical student causing pain to someone else dissipated. Like a ghost, the memory evaporated above my eyes into the pleasant orange light.

"We seem to be doing quite well." It was a new voice. It was difficult for me to move my head, but I could move my eyes. I saw a dark green face mask and horn-rimmed glasses. It was the anesthesiologist.

"Hi, Mac," I said, "I was wondering where you were in all

this turmoil." There was no turmoil. Everything was flowing smoothly, so quietly.

"Things seem to be going quite well," Mac replied, his voice steady and reassuring. There was no variation in pitch, no sign on his part that what I had said had threatened or challenged him. The word "turmoil" simply bounced off him as gently as a soap bubble off a tile wall in the bathroom.

"We are almost ready to go now."

"Any time you say," I replied. I was trying to be light and gay, perhaps even funny, but it did not work. To be honest, my thoughts were not on Mac. I was thinking of that damn Foley catheter, snuggling so neatly down the entire length of the urethra of my penis, and I was saying to myself, "Damn it, I'm going to have a uretheral infection before this damn thing is over! It never fails. You cannot keep those catheters sterile all the time." But I did not want to tell this to him. I was a coward, you see. Mild urethritis could be so easily cared for by either of two antibiotics, and I knew it. It was an hysterical comparison of urethritis to a stenotic coronary artery. I was comparing a splinter in a finger with the amputation of a gangrenous foot.

Why do we think the way we do? To distract ourselves? At that moment I didn't know. Once again I heard the deep, resonant voice of the anesthesiologist. "In a moment, I will inject some fluid into this little vein here, and you will fall asleep, and you will rest quietly, and I'll see you after the operation when you awake." I remember seeing his head, his face turned from me; while I looked at the top of his head, which was covered with a green cap, the two circles of his horn-rimmed glasses snaking from the front of the mask and curling around his ears, I wondered why some men have hair on their ears. "Here we go!" His deep voice reverberating. That was the last thing I recall hearing, seeing, feeling, touching, smelling, sensing, tasting, and breathing — a total silence came to all the senses of my life. No one else's, but my life. I had come to an end at that exact moment.

* * *

It was an extremely different feeling. When you go to sleep, you usually prepare yourself. You say to yourself, "I'm going to

sleep." Your mind wanders, thinking about the day, thinking
about tomorrow, thinking about your little worries. The mind
hopscotches around until, I suspect, the brain simply says to itself, "Enough of all these thoughts; let's put them aside until
tomorrow." And so we sleep. We seem to know that we are
sleeping. We have dreams associated with sleep. We are easily
awakened, various comforts and discomforts reach us, but it is
nevertheless sleep. Now it is a distinctively different feeling to
be anesthetized. It is extremely rapid. You know it's coming at
you. You're told by your anesthesiologist that this colorless
fluid that he is injecting into the tube goes into a vein in the
back of your arm. Like a magic potion, it takes you and sweeps
you from all consciousness. He is going to do the control-
ling. You're not going to dream. You are going to be unconscious. Now that is not sleeping. That is unconsciousness. There
is no texture; there is no smell; there's no feel; no memory.

It is, simply, total unconsciousness of all senses. That is pri-
marily what happens when one is anesthetized. I am talking
about the routine administration of sodium pentothal, which is
injected into the vein to make you unconscious.

Now after the first stage when you become unconscious,
there follows a highly technical stage when the anesthesiologist
decides what sort of gas to use to keep you anesthetized, how
much oxygen to supply you with, how long you're going to be
unconscious. Every anesthesiologist who takes your life as his
responsibility must face a multitude of questions that require
years of training and experience. Anesthesiologists tend, as a
group, to be on the quiet side. They also tend to be very knowl-
edgeable and keenly aware of keeping that body alive. The surgeon, with his knives and probings and sewing, is doing all the
necessary things to you. That is his responsibility. The anesthesiologist keeps your body functioning and alive while it is
being worked on — that is magic.

The coronary bypass seems so simple in principle that
it is amazing that it has taken the medical profession so many
years to perfect it. If there is a clog in a tube and the contents of the tube cannot flow adequately, one simply takes
another tube and attaches one end above the clog and the
other end below the clog. This is basically the entire operation.

Reconstructing the operation, I can see in my mind how this all worked. Now, it's necessary to know that Dr. Shore had said he was going to use the internal mammary artery and attach it to my left anterior descending coronary artery below the point of stenosis. It sounds simple, doesn't it? And since it's an artery, the replacement would expand and contract like the original: Arteries contain small amounts of muscle-like tissue that rebound with each heartbeat; veins do not have that elasticity. For the internal mammary artery to be used, it would have to have a specific diameter, so that it could carry the blood supply to the heart muscle, past the point of its potential clogging. Just in case, since the size could be wrong, the saphenous vein, which runs down the leg from the groin to the ankle, is also removed.

Unconscious, I lay on the table. A team consisting of Dr. Shore and two other surgeons awaited a signal from the anesthesiologist to begin. He nodded to Dr. Shore that I was prepared for surgery. An incision was made along the inside of my leg from my ankle to a point below my knee, and the saphenous vein was dissected away from the tissue lying just beneath the skin. The tributaries were cut and sewn, and the vein, almost twelve inches long, was removed and placed in a sterile solution to await the time when it could be used.

Next, Dr. Shore made an incision through the skin from a point where the two collarbones end, that is, in the center of the breastbone, or sternum, straight down to the end of the sternum above a small cartilagenous ending known as the xiphoid. The incision having been made, blood vessels were tied off, and the sternum was exposed. A rotary saw was used to cut through the bone. Very carefully, the entire sternum was cut exactly down the center. The sternum was then spread apart with retractors so that the heart could be seen contracting.

Now it was necessary to insert a cannula, another tube, into the inferior vena cava and the superior vena cava. These are the largest veins that bring blood back to the heart from the body. It was time to hook my blood supply to the heart-lung machine. The venous blood, which contains the waste products and carbon dioxide picked up from the tissues of the body, is brought to this machine. The carbon dioxide and waste products were removed, and oxygen was restored to the bloodstream. Then another tube from this machine entered the largest artery of the body, the aorta; the heart itself was bypassed and the surgeon could work on it while the body was fed the oxygenated blood necessary for sustaining life.

Meanwhile, the anesthesiologist had inserted a tube down the windpipe into the lungs so that a machine could breathe for me, keeping the lungs open, filling with air, and then collapsing, so that carbon dioxide would be removed from the lungs during surgery. A clamp closed off the aorta below the cannula coming from the tube of the heart-lung machine and carrying oxygenated blood that was pumped by machine through the body.

Dr. Shore touched the heart muscle with a small electrode; the heart stopped its pumping action and began to fibrillate. This means that the muscle fibers of the heart, instead of contracting in a pumping motion, begin quivering mildly so that the surgeon can work on the heart without its being in constant pumping action. (A new technique is being used now called cardioplegia. A solution of potassium is injected and the heart muscle stops all movement, making it easier for the surgeon to operate). Dr. Shore then cut through a membrane called the pericardial sac and held the life-sustaining organ in his hands. He could feel the left anterior descending artery and could pinpoint the position of the clogged portion of the vessel simply by touch. It was hard and not as elastic as the vessel above or below the clogged portion. He examined all the other vessels, the coronary arteries that supply both the right and left ventricles, and felt for different vessels to make certain that they were elastic to his touch and that there was no hardness under his fingertips. But as he felt around both the front and the back of the heart, he noticed that the circumflex artery, which comes directly off the aorta to supply a portion of the heart muscle, had the beginning of a plaque formation that might cause problems five to ten years in the future.

Now he had found two areas of the coronary arteries that had to be bypassed. The other arteries on the right side seemed to be open and in good condition. Since the saphenous vein had already been removed, it was necessary to check the internal mammary artery, which runs along the left side as well as the right side of the sternum, with tributaries feeding the intercostal muscles (the muscles between the ribs). He noticed that the diameter of the internal mammary was satisfactory. He decided to use the artery to bypass the clogged portion of the left anterior descending coronary artery and to use the saphenous vein removed from my leg to bypass the clog that was beginning in the circumflex artery.

The internal mammary artery was pulled away from the chest wall and then attached to the left anterior descending coronary artery, bypassing the closure of this particular artery, which amounted to almost 90 percent. Carefully, Dr. Shore checked the flow of blood through this artery into the coronary and, satisfied, he completed the sewing of the internal mammary into the coronary artery. It was observed for any leakage, and none appeared to be there.

Now the saphenous vein was removed from the sterile solution and examined carefully. There were no difficulties with the openings, and the diameter of the vein was acceptable. It was used to bypass the small closure beginning in the circumflex artery. Once again, Dr. Shore checked the flow of blood through the vein and looked for any bleeding at the points of its incision into the circumflex artery. There was no bleeding and everything seemed to be going well.

Now the pericardial sac was sewn back together, and the wire was placed against the sac on top of the ventricle. A small hole was made between the ribs at this level with the wire coming out of the chest wall. A hypodermic syringe was attached to this wire and taped to my chest wall. This wire lying on the heart and coming out of the chest wall could be attached, if necessary, to a pacemaking machine to regulate the heart beat. Two tubes were now inserted into the pleural cavity (which contains the lungs), their openings placed between the lower ribs. These tubes were used, one on each side, to drain any excess fluid or blood that should have entered the pleural cavity. They were attached to drainage bottles so that the fluid could be observed for signs of possible bleeding and to prevent the accumulation of any fluid that would interfere with my breathing after surgery.

Now I had three openings in my chest wall: one for the pacemaker and two for the tubes draining the fluid from the pleural cavity. Dr. Shore checked everything once again; everything now seemed to be in order. The heart was once again touched with the electrode, and the fibrillation changed to the strong contraction of a normal heart beat. The cannulas were removed from the inferior and superior vena cava and from the aorta, and my heart then began pumping on its own. I was no longer on the heart-lung machine. Dr. Shore examined the beating muscles and felt with his fingers that the blood was travelling through the bypasses he had placed. Satisfied that all was well, he removed the retractors that had kept the sternum open, and used strong wire to sew the two cut edges of the sternum together. The wires held the sternum in place and made certain that the edges were approximated so that they will heal together in a normal fashion. Satisfied with that procedure, Dr. Shore sewed together the muscles that had been cut, and then the skin was drawn together approximately and also sewn.

The right leg, where the saphenous vein had been removed, was checked again. Satisfied that that area was cared for, Dr. Shore then checked the draining tubes coming from the lungs. He informed the anesthesiologist that he was finished. A tube was still down my throat, going into my lungs, and a machine was still breathing for me. Now a large-bore hypodermic needle was inserted into the subclavian artery (which travels along the collarbone on the right side); the needle was attached to an intravenous fluid that contains heparin, a substance that prevents clotting of the blood. This needle has a two-way stopcock so that it can be turned, a syringe being inserted into one of the openings of the stopcock, to extract blood in order to check the amounts of oxygen and carbon dioxide in my bloodstream.

Surgery is now completed. I have had two bypasses, and I am wheeled into the Intensive Care Unit.

Time has no significance while you are under anesthesia. At one moment you are asleep, without feeling, without thought, and the next moment you become aware and have certain sensations.

There is a tube down my throat. It feels the size of a watermelon. I am ravenously thirsty; I feel dehydrated. I also know that I cannot talk. Conclusion reached by this physician, flat on his back in the recovery room: he has an endotracheal tube that is doing the breathing for him. How long I am aware of this feeling is difficult to say, but my guess would be that it was of extremely short duration. Eyes opened. The Roman Colosseum had not changed. The orange lights had not changed. There were figures, nurses, around me; they had not changed. I could not talk; that was a change. I had difficulty in swallowing; that, too, was a change. I seemed to be very dry-mouthed; a third change. I think I fell asleep.

It was different from closing my eyes and being anesthetized, because as I slept I was conscious of sounds: the sounds of gasses going in and out of the tube in my mouth, and the rather garbled sound of nurses and doctors discussing something I could not quite follow at that moment. But it was different. It was sleep, but not the way it was before — unconscious. I can't recall how long I remained this way. After what seemed a very short time, I opened my eyes, and there stood beside me the male nurse whom I called Joe. He looked down at me; I could see his eyes clearly. "How are you doing, Doc?" he asked.

Now you cannot answer with an endotracheal tube down your throat (it still felt to me like something the size of a watermelon). I tried to swallow some saliva. I had no way to tell him that I would have loved a drop of liquid to grease my tongue's movement along the tube inserted down my throat. He seemed to read my mind, however, and he gave me the tiniest chip of ice, a sliver; it slid down my throat. He gave me another. I slept on and off, and each time I awoke there he sort of tucked another sliver of ice into the side of my mouth. I can't recall the duration of time during this episode. It passed smoothly. There is no watch, no clock in view. Joe, the nurse, wears a wristwatch; I try to look at it but I could not see what time it was. Was it daytime? Nighttime? Afternoon? Dawn? There are no windows in the recovery room.

Finally, I wasn't falling back to sleep anymore. I noticed myself getting a trifle irritated at the watermelon-sized tube that remained inside my throat and at the hissing of gas reverberating in every sinus of my skull. I recall not closing my eyes too often. I watched people move about me — Joe or other nurses and several doctors who removed the sheet over my chest and examined something that I could not yet see at that time.

That was my surprise for later. Everything seemed to be going well. I sensed that they were pleased, and that was very reassuring. Behind the masks I could not see their complete expressions, but I could see their eyes and the muscles around their eyes, which expressed what they were feeling.

I don't know how long this period lasted. As I mentioned, time had no essence, no sense, no way to compare. A familiar face appeared; it looked like the anesthesiologist. He spoke, and I knew it was he. He said, very gently, "Well, things are working out very nicely. Joe and I are going to remove this small tube from your mouth."

"Small tube!" I wanted to shout. "This huge, tree-trunk-sized tube, this redwood! Is there anything else you were going to leave in?" Of course, none of this could be verbalized.

Quickly, the tube came out of my mouth, and I remember that first moment, breathing deeply on my own. When I tried to swallow, everything was dry; I said my first word: "Water." Again, my generous nurse supplied me with several slivers of ice that moistened my throat enough to keep me from complaining further. I was without this giant tree trunk of a hose blocking my throat. Now feeling some of my oats, I felt, frankly, irritable and quite bitchy and wanted to let somebody know how unhappy I was. But each time slivers of ice slid down my throat, my irritability was gone. You see, I was very easily placated. Sleep came, and this time without the apprehension that existed before, when I felt the endotracheal tube. It was more of a restful, pleasant, non-apprehensive type of sleep. My eyes closed and I slept.

It wasn't till later, and again I cannot tell you whether it was minutes or hours, that I became aware of the nurses who were flocking around me checking, re-checking, making notes, injecting some pain-killer, some narcotic into my intravenous tubing, which would set me off on a euphoric trip that diminished the pain and mostly diminished my apprehension.

Later, when I was becoming rather alert and conscious of what was going on, I commented to the nurse that the Foley catheter certainly had been in long enough and should be removed. Strange how we attach significance to something within our brain. Perhaps it was a castrating threat to me. I am not too certain. I would prefer to think that the catheter was going to cause future problems and be a source of irritation. I have spoken to other patients about this reaction, and many of them concurred. Perhaps, because they did not go through the years of psychoanalysis that I did, their castration anxiety was on the surface: often they reported the terrifying impression that when the catheter would be removed, their penis was going to be pulled or torn and mutilated in such a way that it would remain on the edge of the catheter. However, I am glad to say, such an incident has never been reported in any medical study.

Six

Struggling out of Intensive Care

I spent three days in the intensive care unit. In the beginning it seemed as if I did nothing but sleep. Occasionally I would awake and find Carol sitting beside my bed holding my hand. Then I would close my eyes again, and when I opened them she was gone.

Hours passed quickly the first day, and I was feeling more alert and aware of my surroundings. The ICU had no windows, and the only way I could tell the passing of time was by a new nurse's face, indicating that another eight-hour shift had begun.

Joe appeared. I asked him how long I had been sleeping, and he said about fourteen hours. Although I felt some discomfort in my chest, it was not entirely unbearable, considering the trauma to the chest wall.

"How would you like to take your first walk?" Joe asked.

"Now?"

"Nothing like the present," Joe replied. "Besides we don't want you staying in bed without moving around. It's one way we can help you avoid pneumonia."

I agreed reluctantly, assuming that Joe knew what he was doing and that it would be best for me to follow the instructions

laid out by the staff. Joe disconnected the wires of the electrodes on my chest leading to the electrocardiogram that was
sitting on a shelf above and behind my bed. There were three
electrodes: two on the left chest wall and one on the right. He
helped me sit up with my feet dangling over the side of the bed.
Then he placed a pair of white knee-length stockings on my legs.
They felt tight and snug.

"What's that?" I asked.

"Like support hose," he answered. "Keeps the blood from
accumulating in the legs. Remember, you have one piece of vein
missing, and the circulation has not formed tributaries to take
up the slack in your extremities. These stockings prevent the
accumulation of fluid in the tissue so that your legs don't swell."

His explanation did it all for me. He had answered all my
unasked questions.

I was still attached to an intravenous feeding and the bottle
hung from a pole. The catheter was still in place draining into a
plastic container. Joe helped me stand, and, carrying the urine
container and another container that caught the fluid from the
tubes draining my pleural cavity, I began to walk. Joe pushed
the pole with the intravenous fluid still dripping into my arm.
This is the way we walked around the room. I was wearing the
typical hospital gown that tied in the back, and I could feel the
breeze up my thighs with each step. We traveled the circum-
ference of the room one time and then Joe brought me back to
bed. He hooked the wires back to the electrodes and I stretched
out in bed, feeling as though I had performed a most arduous
and exhausting task. I felt tired after my first walk, and yet
I was surprised that my body had been able to function so
well just a few hours after open-heart surgery. It amazed and
pleased me. I slept again.

The Bird Man arrived and I used the machine as directed. It
was a little painful to distend my lungs with the necessary air,
but I felt more comfortable after I had used the respiratory
machine.

About two hours later, Joe suggested we do our "traveling
dance" once again, so we started to circumnavigate the room.
This time I saw Vinnie in one of the beds.

"Can we go over and say hello?" I asked Joe.

"I don't think it would be wise. He's still sleeping and

you can see the endotracheal tube is still in place. Let's keep walking. When he's awake we'll visit."

I followed Joe around the room, glad that Vinnie was with me now in the ICU.

Sleeping seemed to be my chief activity during this time. Occasionally blood would be drawn for some chemical tests, but I became so innured that sometimes I was not aware of the needle's puncture; often it seemed as though I had slept through it all. With every passing hour I seemed to gain more strength. In the beginning I traversed the ICU only once or twice, but as each day passed, I was able to walk more comfortably. My breathing distressed me considerably but I did feel more at ease with the precious gas replenishing the oxygen I had used up during my small exercise.

On the second day, when I awoke I saw Vinnie standing before me. "Hi, Doc!" he exclaimed. "I'm walking!"

I smiled at him and told him the next time I would race him around the ICU and the loser had to stay in the ICU an extra day. Sometimes we would meet as we walked around the room, but the nurses wanted us walking and not talking. A wave of a free hand was a sufficient sign of recognition.

Vinnie looked funny with his big ass sticking out of the short hospital gown. When I mentioned it to him, he became a little self-conscious, but we both got a laugh out of this. It hurt when I laughed, but it helped break the monotony of the routine.

Almost moment by moment, as my strength increased, I became less apprehensive. Everyone encouraged me, and I followed orders, leaving my life in their hands. On the third day, Dr. K., an associate of Dr. Shore, came in and told me that it was time to take the tubings out of the pleural cavity. I looked at him somewhat anxiously.

"Nothing to this," he explained. "Take this sterile square bandage and hold it tight against the opening in the chest wall where the tube is protruding." I did as he suggested and watched as he gripped the edge of the tube; in one swift yank the tube was pulled from my chest. Then we repeated the procedure on the other side.

I looked at my chest now. The holes in my chest where the tubing had been were now covered by small squares of gauze.

I had thought that the tubes were a few inches in length, but now I saw them on the tray beside my bed: they were at least ten inches long. I did feel better now that they were removed. I seemed to breathe better.

"How about another walk?" Joe asked.

"I just walked," I protested.

Joe glanced at his watch and smiled. "That was three hours ago."

It was difficult to pick my body up from a sitting position. Joe helped and I swung my legs around and stood up. I was now wearing the supportive hose all the time, in bed as well as out. I was going to wear them the remainder of my stay in the hospital and even at home for several weeks.

Joe and I made our tour of the ICU. This time we seemed to be doing quite a bit of walking and I was amazed at the strength that was slowly returning to my body. When I returned to bed, Joe did not hook up the EKG wires as he had done each time in the past.

"The EKG wires, Joe," I said.

"You're going up to your room now," Joe answered.

"So soon?" I asked.

"You've been here three days and you have been doing extremely well."

I wasn't sure that I wanted to go. Some apprehension swept over me. I liked the nurses and technicians around me. I felt safe that everything was being watched and that all the chemistry and EKG tracing were constantly observed. What would happen in my room? There wouldn't be this constant attention. I wanted to protest, but knew it would not be appropriate. I leaned back in my bed and tried to calm myself and simply accept their decision.

Carol arrived and I told her the "good news," but my face revealed my feelings.

"Don't you know that you're doing so well?" she asked.

"So they tell me."

"Then why the face?" she asked.

I began to explain my apprehension, but she interrupted, asking what I thought was going to happen when I got home. I didn't answer. Going home? I didn't want to think about it.

I thought about some patients that I had treated, and, recalling their apprehension about leaving the hospital when the treatment had been completed, I developed an insight into how they must have felt. I would never dismiss a patient's protestations as lightly as I had in the past.

Joe came by and told us there was a delay because my room was not quite ready. He rehooked the EKG wires and suddenly I felt comfortable again. I knew I was acting like a child, but I couldn't seem to shake the fear of leaving the protective confines of the ICU.

Vinnie approached the bed, accompanied by his nurse. "I hear you're going back to the room."

"So I'm told," I answered.

The nurse tugged at him so I couldn't tell him about what I felt. Would he feel the same way? I could see Joe across the room, caring for another patient. I felt jealous: He was giving his attention to someone else, and I still needed him. I felt deserted. I knew that the protective confines of the ICU were about to be taken away and that I had to make the adjustment in my attitude. I was being infantile and I had to get over this feeling of dependency.

"OK, Doc, we're all set now." He had brought a wheel chair. I let him disconnect the wires to the EKG and help me into the wheel chair. Another nurse began to wheel me out of the ICU. As we passed Vinnie's bed I waved to him, but he was asleep. I hoped to see him back upstairs in a day or so, too.

Carol was in the room, waiting for me. It was good to see her. She assisted me into bed and made me comfortable. We spoke about the friends and relatives who had called over the past few days. The room was filled with plants and flowers. My apprehension about leaving the ICU was rapidly disappearing; by dinner time I was comfortable and happy to be in my own room and preparing myself for ultimate discharge.

Carol told me that Tony had gone to surgery that morning; Vinnie's wife had told her that he was expected back in his room perhaps the next day. Suddenly I found myself being quiet; the euphoria of returning to the room was passing. For some reason, I wanted to be silent.

"Something wrong, honey?" she asked. "You seem so quiet.

Are you tired? Can I bring you something? Perhaps you'd like to sleep?"

I shook my head and began to weep. I knew that I was probably feeling post-surgical depression. I was happy that the whole mess was over and that all the nurses and doctors seemed to be pleased with the results, yet something was going on inside me that I had never experienced before. At first I thought that I was just glad the whole thing was over, that this was the happy kind of weeping. But, no, it wasn't that at all. I could follow my thoughts as I tried to analyze myself and what was going on inside me.

Approximately two weeks had passed since I had been told in the emergency room that there was something wrong with my EKG. I was under stress every second of the day since then, 60 seconds to the minute, 3600 seconds to the hour, and 24 hours broken up into those seconds. I was also in pain; I don't want to leave you with the impression that it was excruciating, but it was, for me, the first time in all the years of my life that I knew what constant pain was. We have all banged our thumbs with hammers, and bumped our shins into furniture. Now it seemed to me that waiting all those seconds and minutes was simply a natural culmination of what I had gone through. I could see that I was distressing Carol, and I did not know what I could say to relieve her. I couldn't ask her to leave the room, to leave me alone; that would have been a terrible insult to her. Even though I didn't want to say certain things that I was slowly beginning to analyze, and even though I didn't want to say it, I knew I was going to. I share all my thoughts with her; it's a habit of over twenty years' duration. I am not ashamed of emotion and am more amused at certain men who consider being emotional and tender and gentle as being unmasculine. But that is not my nature.

That particular afternoon, after going through the surgery, the pain, the discomfort, I said to her, "Had I known that it was going to be like this, I don't think I would have done it." At that moment I meant it — but only at that moment. When that moment had passed, I no longer meant it. I knew that if I had to go through the surgery again, I would. And if I had to go through it three times, I would.

I mentioned to Carol the story of her aunt whom we had

visited in Florida: It had been late May, and the temperatures had been in the very high eighties, she had had a heater blasting away in her sitting room. It had been difficult to find a way to ask her to turn it off, because she had sat wrapped up in a very heavy woolen sweater, her feet curled up near the heating machine. I jokingly had said to her that we northerners had no appreciation for the weather; coming from Connecticut, I found the weather delightfully warm. Since she had been living in Florida for so many years, she was able to feel the chill.

She had given me rather a surprising answer. "You know, I am in my late eighties, and if it takes all this heat to keep me feeling alive, then I trust you will bear with me. Each day is so precious to me that I do not want to relinquish one moment of my life."

Now I understood what she had meant. Life was very precious to her, and if the room was too hot for me, I could leave. I stayed with her, bearing the heat. At the end of the story, I said to Carol, "That's the way I feel now."

It was only two minutes since I had said I would not go through this experience again, yet now I was saying I was going to cling to life more than I had ever done before. I was going to make it. I was going to do all the exercises I had to do and take all the horrible-tasting medicines I had to take, and I was going to get over feeling sorry for myself. I was not going to be a burden to myself.

And all this I poured upon my wife; I drenched her. I could see that although what I had said before had upset her, what I was saying now was acceptable to her. Then I said to her, "You know, when you're under anaesthesia for so many hours, your brain gets sort of cooked a little bit, I think, and you don't remember anything too well." She reached over and held my hand, and we sat quietly. In a moment, I was asleep.

And I dreamt of Connecticut dogwoods and the smell of a freshly cut lawn, in the distance the barking of a dog. The tranquil dream of what I thought was health permeated every aspect of my being.

Seven

I'm No Longer Immortal

I awoke. It was dark outside. The fog in my thinking seemed to have disappeared. My emotions were no longer debilitated by depression. It seemed strange that it had left as fast as it had appeared. Analyzing the past hours, I concluded that it had been simply a post-surgical effect. I recalled reading that patients who go through open heart surgery frequently develop bizarre emotional symptoms. They are distressing both to the patient and to the staff, but they do not last.

I was not tired. I realized that I had slept for a good part of the previous day and most of this night. My eyes were wide open. I was not intoxicated this evening with any sleep-inducing medication or pain-killing substance, so two very important sense organs—my eyes and my ears—and my thinking ability were all tuned in extra fine. I definitely had pain. Touching my chest, I felt that all the electrodes going to the EKG machine were still attached. I worried that in my sleep I might dislodge them while moving, but I knew that if they were, the nurse in the hall would see the changes on the EKG machine that faced her in front of her desk. As my fingers ran along my chest, I felt the wire that was to be used as a pacemaker in case of an emergency.

63

When I turned the lights on, I saw the electrodes and the pacemaker wire that was wound around a five-cc syringe and held in place against my chest with adhesive tape. I was pretty well wired for any physical contingency, considering what was going on inside me. I still had my thoughts, my private self. No one was going to read thoughts skipping along as little waves on the oscilloscope. These were all mine.

I had several alternatives at that moment. I could push the switch that turned on the television set across the room; I had another switch for pleasant, schmaltzy music. I decided against both since I was feeling both bored and wide awake. If I turned on the TV, perhaps I would have seen some ridiculous late show (or maybe even one not so ridiculous — perhaps a Marx Brothers movie); that would have given my sutures a jolt or two if I laughed, so I was not going to chance that. I really did not want to be simply distracted; music in no way appealed to me. In truth, I really wanted to be, for the first time, undrugged, alone with my thoughts.

This was a very private time for me. I knew the nurses were outside, but in the confines of my room I was involved with my thoughts. I had been thinking about my own mortality; at first, the thought had gently nudged my mind as it were, when I was no longer heavily drugged. Occasionally, the thought would come up against me with real ferocity and sort of punch me, making itself known, asserting that it was not simply going to go away.

I don't know how long the feeling persisted. It was the fourth day after my bypass operation, so certainly it wasn't very long in duration. During moments of consciousness the thought was persistent and hung in there. I sort of liked the idea that it was persistent and not to be dismissed so lightly. I had to give it the attention it merited before I could proceed to other thoughts.

Mortality.

Before this experience I don't think I ever gave that word any concern. Now, mortality kept insinuating itself into all aspects of my picture of the future. It was dreadful. I also knew that this thought, which was now conscious, had been the cause of my depression the day before. I hadn't understood it until that moment as I lay quietly in bed in the middle of the dark night. I never had thought about my own death before. I simply had lived my days one after the other. In my eyes, I was immortal. I had proceeded from one day to the next, doing my work, socializing, absolutely sure that there would always be time to do what I wanted, when I wanted to do it. If I didn't feel like writing a scientific paper for publication, well — I would get to it some time in the future.

Was there a future for me now? I had had the operation and everyone was happy with the results. Had it actually extended my life? No one gives guarantees, especially in medicine.

I found myself thinking of all the things I had wanted to accomplish. Strangely, I began to sort out these desires and set up priorities for my life. But where would I begin? The enormity of the decisions overwhelmed me. Now, as these priorities arranged themselves in my mind, I found myself with a problem that I couldn't cope with in that dark room. If ever there was a reason for depression, it was at that moment. I needed time. How much time did I have left? I became irritated at the constancy of thinking about my mortality. I abhorred the whole idea. I will procrastinate no longer on the subject. I had promised myself the exact opposite a moment ago. It's time for the Marx Brothers, I told myself. Besides, I noted, I had to urinate. I rang for the nurse.

In a few moments the door to my room opened and the nurse walked in. Most nurses have similar characteristics. I am not talking about their physical appearance, of course, but about their behavior patterns and the way they perform the job of nursing. It's like seeing a thousand dolls lined up on a shelf; they may look alike in certain aspects, and may all say "Mama" and blink their eyes the same way, but if one takes the time to look carefully, one will see that little unique difference that sets them apart from each other. So, even though I say they are plastic, the same, it is only in the sense of the uniformity of action, performance, and dress. However, this evening nurse was not typical. She was extremely obese, weighing more than two hundred pounds, yet she had a face that was pleasant, a voice that was inquisitive, instructive, gentle but firm.

"You are not asleep," she said.

"I slept most of the day. Perhaps I'm slept out. Why aren't you asleep?" I jested. "It must be rather late."

She laughed and said she was a night person. One of the reasons she went into nursing was to take a job that she would like and enjoy, and she knew no better shift for her than the one she now had from eleven to seven in the morning.

She asked whether I would like a sleeping pill. I declined. "You seem to be so wide awake. Is there something troubling you?" she asked.

I said, "Not really. I am wide awake because I am working out one of those problems of living that every one of us must go through, considering all this business about one's heart."

She chuckled (it was the sound of little bells) and said, "I don't think you have much to be concerned about. That is about your heart. You seem to be doing very well. In fact, excellently."

I felt pleased at hearing those reassuring words; "Thanks, I needed that," I said, imitating a TV commercial. She was about to turn and leave when I stopped her. "Would you mind handing me that duck?" I asked, pointing to the urinary container sitting at the far edge of the room.

She looked at me, and in the dim light I could see a tight firmness shaping her mouth. "We do not use the duck," she said to me. "We go to the bathroom."

Now if there is one thing that gets me simply in an uproar, it is the use by a professional of the pronoun *we* when *you* is meant. "How are 'we' today?" "What are 'we' going to have for lunch today?" That *we* simply arouses the worst kind of response in me. I said to her, "If 'we' do not get that duck, 'we' will urinate in the bed."

Now, we were locked in combat. She was physically stronger, but I had made a judgment that I was intellectually superior. Her reply to my comment was, "If 'we' urinate in the bed, I will have to change the sheets. And when I change the sheets, you will be rolled from side to side. It will be excruciatingly painful for you to go through the process of having your sheets changed while you are in bed. Do 'we' understand what 'we' are saying?"

I looked at her, and for some time said nothing. Quickly, I reviewed the alternatives. What options were open? I could obstinately attempt to reach that duck sitting at the other side of the room, but I knew that getting up into a sitting position would be exceedingly painful because of the wires that were hanging around my chest, sending out those interminable beeps of my EKG to the oscilloscope on that nurse's desk, and my energy level would have been rated about zero. For me even to sit up, I would have needed her cooperation and assistance. So, option one was rejected: I could not reach for that urinary container.

Option two, I could simply relax and urinate in bed like a child who knows better but is too lazy, perhaps too frightened, or simply genetically eneuretic. Again, however, to urinate in the bed and wet the sheets, I would have had to go through the rather difficult and painful remaking of the bed. To change the sheets with me out of bed, she would have had to help me stand up and get out of bed, but she had threatened to remake the bed with me in it. That was a dirty trick, I thought.

So, option three, looking her directly in the eyes, I said, "Won't you give me a hand and help me out so I can get to that damn bathroom?"

Her hand came forward, and chuckling again she said to me, "We made a wise decision."

"I *think* we made a wise decision," was my answer. I would have liked to laugh with her, but it was still a bit painful to laugh; even the slightest chuckle caused discomfort. She helped me into the bathroom.

Strange thing about the bathroom. The bowls that were built into the hospital seemed very high. I had the feeling of sitting on the bowl with my feet just barely touching the floor; that is how high the toilet seemed to me. I waited for an eternity for the stream of urination to start; ultimately, it came. That damn Foley catheter had irritated me in some way, making it difficult now to start to urinate. Having finished, I pulled up the bottoms of my pajamas and walked back slowly into the dimly lit bedroom, I found that my nurse had made her departure. It appeared that "we" did not need her anymore. I very slowly and cautiously climbed back into bed, put my head onto the pillow, and decided that I had exercised enough for the day. I retreated into a more desirable state: sleep.

The noise and movement of a nurse bringing in my breakfast tray awakened me. It was daylight, and Carol was sitting in
the chair against the window. She had been waiting for me to
awaken.

"Did you sleep well?" she asked as she helped me sit up.

I was staring at the breakfast tray, not knowing where to
start, so she took over. She placed the cup of orange juice into
my hand. As we spoke, she handed things to me, deciding what
I was to eat and the order I was to eat them in. I was truly
appreciative. She shared a cup of coffee with me. I told her
about my "combat" with the night nurse. The story seemed to
amuse her a great deal; she commented upon my own attitude
about patients who do not follow instructions: if they don't
follow instructions, why bother to treat them?

"It was the principle of the thing," I said.

"It was the obstinacy of the thing," she replied.

In the silence that followed, I had the feeling she was waiting for me to say something. I wanted to tell her about my
reflections on death; perhaps she had had similar thoughts
while she had been alone at night. Finally, I said to her, "I
found myself awake. I didn't know what time it was, but it
was dark, I remember. And I wondered what would have happened, had I not come back from surgery, had I not made it
so to speak — well, damn it, you know what I mean — had I
died."

Her response was, "You have such a delicate way of describing your feelings."

"But it's true," I replied. "I was thinking of my mortality."

"And what did you conclude?" she asked.

"Oh," I said, "not very much. I thought to myself, 'I'm
no longer immortal.'"

"Were you immortal a month ago?" she asked while gazing
at me over the rim of the coffee cup.

"I never thought too much about it. Took it for granted.
That was why I was so depressed yesterday. Except it was unconscious. Now I'm quite aware of it all."

"Did you think you were someone special?"

"Frankly, yes," I answered.

"Terrible discovery," Carol replied.

"Very funny. Do you think about those things?"

"No. I take it for granted. Ever since I learned what the word meant."

"I'm trying to be serious," I said. I opened the container of Gelusil and gulped it down. "At least I won't get a stress ulcer." Next came the potassium; I held my nose as I swallowed the fluid.

"Vinnie came up to the floor yesterday, late afternoon," Carol said. "Eleanor drove with me this morning to the hospital. She's with him now. Vinnie told her that Tony developed some high temperature and was placed on a refrigerated mattress to bring his temp down. I wonder how he's doing."

Suddenly the door burst open and Vinnie's wife, Eleanor, rushed in.

"Vinnie won't let me into the room. He said I'm bringing germs!" she exclaimed. "What should I do? The nurses said this is common and that some patients act funny when they come back from the ICU."

I looked at Carol and smiled. If it wasn't depression, it could be some other mental reaction. "Stay here, I'll go speak to him," I said.

I gingerly got out of bed, put my bathrobe on, and walked to Vinnie's room. He was finishing his breakfast. I sat in the chair next to his bed.

"How're things going?" I asked. "You look great."

"Tired," he said. "When are Eleanor and Carol coming?"

I said they were both in my room and told him what Eleanor had said.

"Oh, God, did I say that?" he asked. I stood up and told him that I would send Eleanor back.

"Besides, there are germs everywhere. In fact, I must have dragged a few in just now." Vinnie looked at me quizzically. I was certain he did not recall anything he had said in the past few minutes. "Enjoy your potassium," I said.

"Thanks," he replied. "It tastes awful."

I returned to the room and sent Eleanor back to Vinnie.

"Some psychiatrist," Carol said.

I snapped my fingers. "Easy," I said. "Let's go for my morning constitutional."

Eight

The Eiffel Tower in Milwaukee

Now a routine began and continued until the day I left the hospital. The daily sponge bath was followed by breakfast, which was usually the same: it consisted of juice, cereal with skimmed milk, or dry cereal with sliced bananas (bananas are high in potassium, and I still needed the potassium that had been depleted by using the heart-lung machine). I was allowed decaffeinated coffee or tea. Carol and I would read the newspaper, and then I would begin my exercises. I did not exactly walk at a snail's pace — but close to it. I would try to keep walking for at least ten minutes and then rest. Yes, I huffed and puffed, and anyone could have blown me over, but I persisted, and each day I was able to walk another minute more; finally, I worked up to about twenty minutes. Each time I would try to walk faster, increase my pace.

One day the nurse approached and asked whether we would like to try the Eiffel Tower. She led us through an exit door and to the steps; the stairwell went up to the next floor of the hospital. The enormous distance upward seemed to be a climb of one thousand steps. I stood with one foot on the first step, looking for some excuse to return to bed. The nurse stood by silently. Carol hesitated as she reached for my arm and then withdrew it. The signs were all about me. I had to do this myself; no help allowed.

"Remember, Doctor, there is no time limit. Take as much time as you need. Also, coming down is much easier."

"Very cute," I mumbled to myself as I climbed to the second step. Then to the third and fourth. I rested, then took the fifth, and went to the top without a stop. For a moment I thought how much simpler it would have been if they had had bannisters and I had been able to slide down. When I reached the bottom step there was a cheer from Carol and the nurse. I had done it! I held onto the railing for a moment, waiting to catch my breath. I was pleased with myself. I must have been wearing a silly grin.

"Would you like to try it again?" the nurse asked.

"I'll take a rain check," I answered between heavy breaths.

"Are you beginning or ending?" a voice called from the top of the Eiffel Tower. It was George Walcott, the cardiologist assigned to me. He was tall—a beanpole. I envied his trim appearance, his joviality, and most of all his health. Perhaps near forty, he looked more like twenty-one. I watched him descend the steps with his usual bounce and verve. It was always pleasant when he appeared. We all went back to my room, and he quickly wrapped the blood pressure cuff around my arm and took the readings.

"Damn good," he said, smiling. He seated himself on a chair beside the bed and placed his feet on the edge of the bed. George always made me feel better; I liked his direct approach to any of my questions.

"Did you climb the steps without having to stop?" he asked.

"Without a stop," Carol answered for me. She was as pleased as I was.

"Won't be long now," George said. "When you get home it is absolutely essential that you exercise that repaired heart. It's a muscle and it needs exercise."

"When do I go home?" I asked, although I wasn't in any hurry. There was security in the hospital; this question dominated my thinking, because I was not yet that secure.

"Soon," George replied. "A few more days." He rose, pulled out his stethoscope, and listened to my lungs; he brought the bell around to my chest wall and listened intently for a while. "Good. Everything is good."

"George," I asked, "tell me what I have to look forward to when I get home?"

"First, you do as much walking around the hospital as you can. Try to increase the pace of your walk. You may find yourself a little short of wind, but that's all right. You'll know when you've had enough. Just like the Eiffel Tower, you thought it would be impossible, but you did it. Find a flat stretch of road first. Measure the distance of one mile on your car's odometer. Then start doing that mile. Time yourself. Try to decrease the amount of time it took each time you do the mile. Once you feel rather comfortable with the speed and timing, increase the distance to two miles, then three, and try to work yourself up to five miles."

"In Connecticut?" I asked. "The temperature these early January days will be below freezing. I thought cold air was harmful."

"Nonsense," he said. "You'll bundle up; wrap a scarf around your mouth and nose if it's that cold. Beside cold air carries more oxygen than warm air."

"My son bought a stationary bicycle. I suppose I could use that if it snows badly."

"Sure," George said, "but the exercise is not just for your legs. You want to expand your chest muscles and move your arms. If you have a YMCA or a gym of some kind nearby, it would be better. Swimming and walking are the preferred exercises for the next three months."

"When do I go back to work? Not that I'm that eager for it now."

"When you get home, see your internist. He'll still have to check your clotting time, because you're taking an anticlotting drug. He'll be better able to advise about work. Remember, Joe, you'll also be seeing your cardiologist, and he will set up a stress test for you some time in the future. Let these two men guide your decisions about work. And also, no stress!"

No stress, I said to myself. How does one accomplish that miracle? When I had returned from the stay in Stamford Hospital before surgery, they had given me Valium; that had knocked me out completely. I had seemed to be in a haze all day, and the marvelous thing was that I had seemed to have no stress. In fact, I would describe myself then as a zombie. People had visited, but I had no recollection of their being in the house; Carol had had to remind me that Ron King had been over with the will and the power of attorney and that Dan Konover had been over to make certain that some tax matters had been properly handled.

"I had some Valium and it made me forgetful. Would that be a good tranquilizer?"

"If it works that way, no; it wouldn't let you function. Try a less potent medication. Also, when you get back from work, sometimes a drink helps you relax for a few minutes. A small glass of scotch or some other drink that you like. That is, in moderation: one drink is sufficient."

"I think I like that phase of recovery." I smiled at George, feeling more secure knowing that there was to be no extreme change in my life patterns.

When George had left, I suggested to Carol that we take another walk. This time I felt more energetic, and suddenly I decided to see whether I could make it up and down the Eiffel Tower again. We went to the hallway and I looked at those steps. I knew I had to try it again. Slowly, I climbed the steps to the top without stopping and came down the steps with ease At the bottom I smiled at Carol. "Peacock!" she exclaimed.

We walked to Vinnie's room. Eleanor was sitting with him. We began to talk about going home. I would probably leave first, followed by Vinnie and then Tony. I told Vinnie about George Walcott's advice and we talked about the places we would find at home to walk and exercise. Vinnie belonged to the Italian Center in Stamford; I thought I would join the YMCA. We joked about being allowed only one drink per day; Vinnie said he preferred wine, and since wine had less alcohol he could have several glasses.

I convinced Vinnie to join me; we left our wives to relax

and talk. When we passed Tony's room we found him asleep. We knew he was two days behind us in his recovery and let him sleep. As we walked, we met other patients; soon we had a crowd of five patients walking around the hospital floor. Some of us were breathing heavily, and finally, after fifteen minutes, all of us collapsed in a corner of the wing of the corridor that had a few chairs and sofas to accommodate us.

Three more patients joined us in the alcove. Some of our group had just arrived; still others had been having blood tests and X-rays. We were all at different stages of the bypass procedure. The conversation was rambling and chaotic, and certainly it was nebulous — it didn't seem to be going any place. Everyone had his own anxieties he was trying to deal with; when it came out in conversation that I was a physician, many questions were suddenly directed at me. I tried to be as helpful as possible, but I could not answer their technical questions.

Slowly, the conversation took a different tack. It fascinated me because I had nothing to do with the subject matter — at least in terms of bringing it up — and I cannot for the moment recall actually who started the conversation. I do know that the question began to arise, with great clarity and urgency: what would happen to us all after heart surgery? What would happen to us sexually after heart surgery? Would we be the same as before? I suppose that most of us agreed that it would certainly take time to adjust physically to the new feelings and to the changes within our bodies and, most of all, to adjust emotionally to the changes we were going through.

I am going to make a confession here because even though I am a fairly introspective individual and I certainly had given this whole subject some thought, we had never discussed it openly. I became fascinated with the subject. I tried to recall who brought up the subject. I addressed the group frankly: "Whose subject was this? Did somebody bring this up for any particular reason?" Nobody was willing to admit that he was the first person to suggest the subject and nobody was willing to admit, at least at this time, that it was a problem that we needed to discuss.

The first comment came from Bill. He explained to the

group, "You know, it is not just my heart that has been operated on. You see, I had a heart attack before I came, so I sort of
went through that kind of anxiety before."

One of the other men in the group agreed. "Yes, that's quite
right. I also had a heart attack before. I haven't been operated
on yet, but I can recall this tremendous amount of anxiety about
intercourse."

Then Bill laughed, relieving a great deal of embarrassment
felt by everyone in the group. "You know, if it was just the
heart attack, fellas, I don't think I would have any problems,
because since my heart attack, I have been having intercourse.
It's true. Before I have intercourse, I take a nitroglycerine
tablet, which helps me a greal deal."

Some of the other fellows agreed that they also used this
method.

There was still a number of us who did not quite belong in
the group that had experienced a heart attack, or the group that
had had to take a nitroglycerine tablet as a prophylactic measure
before intercourse. We were in a stage of not really knowing. I
know I certainly was part of the inexperienced group. I, in addition, had no history of angina, although many of the others did.
But as we began to talk about the subject (rather heatedly I
may add), everybody had to admit that this was one subject
that distressed him deeply. It was a subject that they found
almost impossible to discuss with their physicians, and it
was equally difficult to discuss it with their wives. The next
revelation shocked me (it shouldn't have, since I am often exposed to open discussions) because there were these men who
stated that this was the first time that they had ever discussed
sexual intercourse with anyone, even friends, never mind total
strangers whom they had just met in the hospital.

"What do you think is the reason we are doing this now?"
I inquired.

There was a heavy-set, very tall, well-educated gentleman in
his late fifties who commented that perhaps there were two
reasons, at least for those who had not gone through surgery.
One, they wanted to know whether they were going to live
through surgery. Two, it was much more comfortable to talk

about such a very personal and delicate matter to total strangers who had something in common with each other.

Many others in the group agreed with his comments. A fellow who appeared to me to be the youngest member of the group spoke up. He said he was 32. He had gone to a local YMCA during one of the Cardiac Weeks and after the tests (on a bicycle and then on a treadmill) the cardiologist informed him that there were some changes in his electrocardiogram. One thing led to the other. Ultimately he had an angiogram which revealed three vessels that were involved, and he was scheduled for at least three bypasses in the next few days. "I asked that question, now that we're being frank and open about it. I was being a wise guy, but I turned out to be the biggest fool here." We made amends and tried to make him more comfortable with his self-revelation. I was proud of him because it took great courage for him to be honest and speak frankly on this subject.

"You know, fellas," he continued. "I'm thirty-two. You guys are fifty or in your fifties or sixties. I sort of felt that when you hit fifty, you guys were sort of over the hill and couldn't get it up anymore. I don't know why I got that idea, but I guess it's because I'm ignorant and nobody ever told me any different. But I'll tell you one thing, it certainly makes me feel a hell of a lot better to know that if I live to my fifties and sixties, I'm going to be able to get it up."

The hall reverberated with our laughter, and several nurses came by and tried to inquire as to what was going on. One of the men told them that this was a very private men's meeting, a chauvinistic conversation, and that we would appreciate if the nurses left the group so we could resume our conversation. I suspect that those nurses knew or had an excellent idea about what the boys in the hall were talking about.

When I returned to my room I found myself still thinking about the conversation that we had. I did not think the way they did. I wondered about it. I was the only one not concerned about my sexual performance, but every one of them was. There must be something wrong with me, I thought. To be outnumbered by such quantities, you must come to but one conclusion — that you are the oddball — not the other group.

This subject matter began to get under my skin. I was beginning to be distressed by the whole thing and I found myself dissecting and analyzing and pulling it apart, as if it was some anatomical specimen, making it yield its structure to me in all its aspects. And then slowly it became a little easier for me to see what was happening. I had spent many years in psychoanalysis. I never thought for many years, especially since the end of my analysis, that I had any particular sexual hangups, anxieties or fears about my performance. That had all been dissected and examined and reexamined under the microscope while I was on the psychoanalytic couch. I thought for a moment how snobbish I felt. I had gone through and studied something that none of these gentlemen had. I was unique. But that didn't quite ring true, you see, because one does not need or require years of psychoanalytic treatment to develop in a "normal" (oh, that terrible word) fashion. There are millions of men who have never seen a psychoanalyst's office and who function extremely well, who know their sexual capacities, are not ashamed of their feelings, and have no hangups, anxieties, or fears. They are capable of making love. They are not concerned about their ability to perform. No, that was not the problem circulating among the group in the hall. It was very different. What made us different from ordinary men? Surely, it was that we were at various stages of serious open heart surgery, some preparing for discharge, some recuperating, some just completing surgery, some just up for the first day from ICU, some ready to go tomorrow, some not ready until the day after, some who had just arrived today. Indeed, we were a motley crew, but there was an obvious common denominator.

It still perplexed me. It still annoyed me that all the men were upset, questioning, raising thoughts and ideas and anxieties about sexual performance after surgery. It did not make sense to me that all the others had to be severely neurotic because they had not gone through psychoanalysis.

I went over it again and again, but no reason for their behavior came to me. Well, I thought, why not take a little walk, get one of those fellows, speak to him privately? You're a good psychoanalyst yourself. You can be diplomatic. You could obtain certain information that would be difficult to obtain in a group or a crowd. Now, I don't really say this in a snobbish way. It is really a scientific — at least in my mind — probing of an emotion that confronted a group of men. I walked down the hall, past one room — he was asleep. Another room — I did not think I could reach him. He seemed to be rather retiring, and I didn't think he would be a suitable candidate for the kind of questioning I was interested in. And then there was Frank, the young man who had brought up the question of sexual performance. He was sitting in bed, watching TV. I knocked on his door and asked, "Would you like some company?" He reached over and flipped the switch, turning off the television set, and said, "Sure, Doc, come on in," beckoning with his hand. I entered and sat on the chair on the side of the bed, turned it so that I faced him as he lay on his back. "That was quite a session we had, Doc, wouldn't you say?"

"Yes," I replied. "I was particularly interested in your remarks, though."

"Oh, which ones are you talking about?" he asked. "I made plenty of them out there. I think I must have sounded like a first-class jackass."

"No," I said, "as a matter of fact, you brought out some fears about sexual performance that almost everyone was worried about." I could see him shift his position, not quite certain whether he was going to like this conversation. I didn't want to push him and waited patiently for him to pick up on the clue.

"It's true, isn't it, Doc? Those guys really were worried, just like I was, but I don't think they were worried *as much* as I was."

"Why do you feel you were more concerned?" I asked.

"Well, no offense, Doc, but you know, I'm thirty-two; you guys are in your fifties, maybe one or two in your forties. You see, fucking's mighty important to me. When I hop in the sack, my ass is like a jackhammer."

"But it will be again," I said.

"How the hell do you know?" he asked. "Now I don't mean to be fresh to you, Doc, but how the hell do any of us know? You know, Doc, I even asked my cardiologist who shipped me out here about it. No, that's a lie, Doc; I really didn't ask him, but I tried to ask him. I tried to say, "You know, Doc, would I be as good as I used to be?" But he didn't pick up on my question. If he did, I had the feeling it would make him mighty uncomfortable. I thought if I pushed the topic any further, he, goddamn it, was going to blush."

"Well," I said, "There is no doubt that it is a very important question. I think this is one of the reasons that it puzzled me after our group broke up. Why hadn't this question been answered by someone else, by the cardiologist, by some specialist — or perhaps by someone who had experience."

"Hey, Doc, that'd be a great idea!" he exclaimed. "Imagine having some guy come up here, saying to us, 'You know fellas, this is what it's gonna be like when you're gonna be well; you're gonna get laid again.' But I guess Puritan is Puritan; wouldn't you say, Doc?"

"Well, you do have a point," I replied. "Puritan is Puritan, but Puritan does not have to be stupidity."

"Well," he continued, "you know, Doc, I'm not due for surgery for two days, but I watch you guys who've been down there and come back. I don't know how you were before, because I didn't know you then, but I see you fellas now, and you shuffle. You don't walk down the hall. You know, when I take a walk, I take a walk. My feet are light, I'm dancing. But, Doc, no offense, even *you* shuffle. Your slippers, they rub on the floor like you can't lift them too high. I hope it means this is just the early stage of your recovery."

I had to laugh. "Well, Frank, I sure hope that's all it is. I don't think I would like to be doing the open heart surgery shuffle for the rest of my life."

He swung his body so that he looked into my eyes directly. "The guys out there say you're a psychiatrist."

I said, "Yes."

"Well," he said, "I reckon if anybody knows about sex, you're the expert here."

I replied, "Well, I don't know if I'm the expert. I would say I know a bit more than most."

Frank reached over the edge of the sheet that covered him and played with the corner of it, rolling it around his index finger as he formulated a question that apparently was extremely important to him. "You know, Doc, you had your days; you're twenty years older than I am. I figure you had twenty years more of sex than me. Now I ain't offending you by talking this way to you?"

"No, Frank," I answered, "Not at all."

"What I mean," he continued, "is you've got those years on me. Maybe it's not as important to you. You have other things more important, you know, like raising a family and things, but for me, well, you know. . . I think about it all the time. You know, I work at a mill, big old lumber mill, crappy old place, but you know, come Friday night I feel like I'm ready to explode. I gotta get it. That's what keeps my blood moving all week. I don't think you feel that way, the way I do, Doc."

I remained silent for a moment. I really felt for him. I had felt that way once, perhaps not so often as of late, but I knew what he was talking about. I said to him, "If you give me a chance, Frank, I'm going to try to explain something to you that perhaps will help you understand what is happening to you now. I hope it will also help you understand why you are going through this dilemma just as I'm going through it and all those other guys are going through it."

He sat up in bed, said, "It better be a good explanation, Doc, because I can't believe that when I get in an uproar you guys know and feel what it means to me."

"But they *do* know what it means and feels to you, Frank," I insisted. "Perhaps not as much as you feel it now within your own body, but I assure you they felt it when they were your age and even older. But they felt the same thing, Frank. That's a monopoly I'm afraid you don't possess. But that's a good reason to come to the hospital for the operation, isn't it?"

"Damn right," Frank mumbled.

"You know," I began, "there are two instincts that are most important to man. The first is survival. It drives a man. It pushes him to act in ways that sometimes are shameful, sometimes beautiful, and sometimes absolutely heroic. To do anything you have to to stay alive. Survival is the strongest instinct we possess."

"O.K. That makes sense."

"The second instinct is also very powerful. That is the need for sexual gratification. That's what you are talking about."

"Right," Frank interjected.

"Your sexual instincts cannot be acted upon unless you survive. You must survive so that you can make love. That's why you're having this operation. You'll survive and then you'll make love. Does that make sense?" I asked.

I could see his mind whirling. "Yep," he said, "I know what you mean. You can't use a hard-on if it's attached to a dead brain, eh?"

"Well," I admitted, "it's not a statement that I had ever heard before, but I think it's quite adequate. You're quite right. An erection requires a live brain, a live body, and a *good* heart." I could see his eyes sort of squinting a little, and I sensed that at that particular moment he was going through an abreaction, a reliving of some beautiful, lustful relationship. Feeling intrusive, I tapped him on the foot and said, "I'll see you tomorrow, Frank."

He grunted, "O.K., Doc." His eyes remained squinted.

I shuffled — I must admit that — out of his room and entered my own, removed my bathrobe, and got into bed and I wondered. Someday I'm going to feel better, I thought, and someday I'm going to want to make love, and how am *I* going to feel about it? There was no one for me to get answers from, so, I said to myself, "Excuse me, honey, but tonight I've got a headache." I reached over and turned out the lights. In a moment I was fast asleep.

Nine

Ten Inches of Metallic Snake

Every day Richard Shore visited. After his examination we would chat awhile. He was interested in art and did charcoal sketches as a means of relaxation and self-gratification. I never understood how he kept up with his hectic schedule of surgery. From early morning until late afternoon he operated — and that's not to mention the emergencies that occurred. His energies seemed boundless.

Once I told him that he was a combination of both my sons. Jonathan was a medical student and wanted to be a surgeon; my other son, Charles, was an artist. I tried not to detain him with too many questions. He aroused a protective feeling in me; I would admonish him to rest. Gently, he would smile and continue his examination, only saying that he was pleased with my progress.

On Friday he announced that I would be discharged on Sunday morning. That meant I would have been two weeks to the day in Milwaukee.

"If I have time tomorrow, I'll come by and remove the stitches, but I believe I have surgery tomorrow. If I don't make it, I'll have Dr. K. come by."

I thanked him for everything he had done for me, wanting
him to know my appreciation in the event I would not see him
again. I could not help liking this man!

Saturday arrived. Carol had made the travel arrangements
and had called Ronnie King to pick us up at the airport on
Sunday.

As the morning progressed, friends would come into the
room and we would play a little cards or just shoot the bull.
Around nine in the morning a surgeon appeared. He introduced
himself as Dr. Shore's assistant and asked how things were going.
My friends quietly left the room so that only Carol remained
with us, and we began to talk. Not so much about the operation;
I was more interested in him. How in the world had he arrived
in Milwaukee? What interested him in cardiac surgery? He
looked Indian, Pakistani—I didn't know which. His name
was difficult to pronounce, so I called him Dr. K. He told
me about his experience. He had gone to school in India, but he
had trained at several famous hospitals in America, such as
Charity Hospital at Tulane, later at Chapel Hill in North Caro-
lina, at Michael Reese in Chicago, and at several other institu-
tions before arriving at Milwaukee to assist Dr. Shore. I fig-
ured rather rapidly that he had spent eight years learning
his craft of cardiac surgery and with great pride he considered
his present assignment to be the peak of his career. He didn't
speak explicitly about his past, although he mentioned names of
various prima donna surgeons and the difficulties a foreign
medical graduate experiences in obtaining positions in this
country. Along the way he had been hurt and perplexed, but he
was determined to succeed and continue to learn. Then, suddenly, he changed the subject: "You have been such a good
listener, Doctor, that I am going to do something I haven't done
for some time." I couldn't imagine what he meant. And he said,
"I am going to remove all your stitches. Usually nurses do this,
it's a simple procedure, but I want to have the honor of removing them, so that we can continue our talk."

Now my first inclination was to be pleased and flattered.
My second inclination was the exact opposite. He hadn't done
it in several months; the nurses were probably much more experienced in cutting a suture. But I couldn't offend Dr. K.

I was sure that even though he hadn't done it in several months he still was an expert. He turned to the nurse and asked her to bring in the tray with the scissors, clamps, and all the other necessary paraphernalia to remove all the junk that was still hanging from my chest wall and from my left leg. He slipped on some rubber gloves and bathed the area, very quickly, very accurately, and started on my leg first. Snip, snip. Pull, pull. Snip, snip. Pull, pull. The sutures were pulled through the skin two at a time, until all were removed. How pleasant, I thought, to be free!

"Now, let us take a look at the chest," he said. Once again he bathed the area, sterilizing it. This time the procedure was different; he pulled out each suture after he snipped it and examined the suture line. Was it closed, or was it open? When he was satisfied that the line was still closed, he would repeat the process with the next suture, all the way up the line, through twenty-eight sutures. The skin held together; it did not crack open. He admired the work. "You heal very nicely. You don't heal with thick scarring tissue. A year from now it will be very difficult for people to know you even had surgery."

A year from now! I wouldn't care if it were ten years from now. I didn't care if it would stay forever. This is my badge. I earned it. It made no difference to me if it would remain or disappear. I was proud of my badge.

The only thing left on my chest was the 5-cc syringe with a wire curled inside my chest, approximately between the fifth and sixth ribs. He cut the nylon cord that kept the syringe attached to the skin and pulled the adhesive tape from around the syringe that held it against my chest wall. Then he gently tugged on the string, and the wire kept coming out of my chest. At first an inch, then two, then three, then four, then five. I said to myself, "Oh my God, where has this wire been?" And I realized it had to be someplace near the sinus rhythm pacemaker of my heart, which produces the rhythmic beat of the heart, so that in the event that anything went wrong, the wire could be electronically induced by a pacemaker to pace the heart more regularly.

Then we were up to six inches; then to seven. Mesmerized, I watched as we reached ten inches and the tip of the wire popped out. He held it up, as though it was some fantastic jewel, some priceless piece of metal, as it dangled from the end of the syringe. It hung in the air like a metallic snake.

I said, "I wonder if I may have that. I don't think you intend to re-use it." He agreed, saying, "No, we have no intention of re-using it. You're certainly welcome to it."

I wrapped it in a small surgical towel and handed it to my wife, who throughout the procedure must have been terribly shocked, hypnotized and fascinated with what had gone on in the last few moments. She held the syringe and stretched the wire to straighten it out, as if in her mind she was taking a tape measure to measure a piece of cloth; figuring out the inches, she slowly dropped it back into the surgical towel, and wrapped it, and placed it on the table beside the bed.

"Well, there you are," Dr. K. said. "All ready to leave tomorrow. Dr. Shore sends his regards. He is in surgery at present. He regrets that he will not be able to see you tomorrow either, before you go, because he is also scheduled for surgery tomorrow."

"Will you give him my best regards?" I replied. "Will you also tell him that I'll never forget him? I have no way of ever truly repaying him, but if I meet patients in the future who require bypass surgery I will certainly tell them that he is the best."

Dr. K. simply looked at me, not knowing what to do with this expression of positive transference that I was spouting. In an embarrassed way he began to leave the room, saying, "I'll give him your messages." Silently, he disappeared through the door.

About this time a nurse appeared with lunch; as usual, the food was not exactly the most appetizing one could imagine. My appetite was not that terrific anyway. It didn't mean that much to me one way or another. I nibbled here and there, picked at the food, and made sure I took my medication; Carol helped with the rest of the tray. I lay back and looked at my chest, denuded of all the paraphernalia, wire, and tubes; I looked at the scar and I could feel my chest expanding with each breath I took. I suddenly said to myself, "You know, kid, it's been two full weeks; an awful lot's happened." Carol suggested that perhaps this would be a good time to take a shower instead of a sponge bath, to prepare myself for fresh pajamas, because tomorrow morning we would leave at 10:00 to be at the airport at 11:30.

Now I don't want you to get the idea that I was capable of zipping around the room and playing games. No, I was capable of taking one very short step at a time — not too many steps in a row; I'd be breathing very heavily throughout — thankful, of course, that I *was* breathing. I took my shower, very carefully and slowly, put on my bathrobe, and returned to the room. I stood before the full-length mirror, ready to take the bathrobe off and put the new pajamas on, and I looked at my body. Hairless, except for my head, I looked like a plucked chicken. I looked at my pubic area and suddenly found something gross and hysterically comical.

Carol called apprehensively, "Is there anything wrong?"

I replied, "Do you really want to see something funny?"

"You know," she said, "after two weeks, yes, I would like to have a good laugh."

"Come here," I said. When she stood beside me, I announced, "I am now going to unfold the curtain of my bathrobe. And I want you to look at this body that you have seen a billion times over the past twenty and some odd years. And I dare you not to laugh."

"I don't think there's anything funny in what you are saying," she replied. "And I think that your sense of humor has been completely distorted by the number of hours you've been under anaesthesia."

I flung my bathrobe open, standing before the full-length mirror, and in the reflection I could see her eyes travel from my head down my face, across my chest, then the stitches, and then stop at my pubic region. The smile started slowly, just slightly curled the lip. Then she was no longer in control. Her teeth showed; then her mouth opened, and she was laughing along with me. "How do you like that, baby?" I asked.

She answered, "Oh my God, it looks — please forgive me — but it does look like the neck of a plucked chicken lying in a box in the supermarket. The only thing missing is the cellophane wrapper."

I said, "I can accommodate you very easily. I'll see if I can dig up some cellophane."

Like two children who had shared a *very* private joke, we discussed the aspects of this discovery. Would wax paper be better than cellophane? Could one get one of those little tags that put down the unit price and the weight? How would we weigh this? A gentle knock on the door interrupted this very personal conversation. In walked George, the cardiologist.

"The two of you seem to be in the middle of something. Should I return later?"

I asked him to come in, since the mood had been shattered. He seated himself in his usual chair at the foot of the bed; Carol remained in the chair beside the bed. He had my chart in his hand, and went through it page by page, saying that everything looked fantastic. "I note the stitches and every little thing had been removed from your chest cavity."

I replied, "Amen." I felt fine. He approached me with his stethoscope and blood pressure cuff, took my blood pressure, clucked that it was marvelous, and that my pulse was good, too. He had me sit up in bed, and his cold stethoscope ran up and down my back, while he asked me to breathe in and out through my mouth; he mumbled that my lungs were clear and good. The stethoscope, now just a trifle warmer, was on my chest; George listened to my heart sounds and clucked again that they were good. Then, rolling the blood pressure cuff into a ball to be placed back into the container and taking his stethoscope out of his ears to dangle around his neck, he said, "Looks like everything is under control. I'm going to miss you."

"I'll miss you, too. You have been steady, very reassuring to me. When you were in my room and had examined me with your blood pressure cuff and your stethoscope, I could see you write little notes in the chart on your lap. It was reassuring to me to know that everything was going according to Hoyle, or at least according to George."

He said, "I understand you're scheduled to leave tomorrow."

"Yes," I replied, "We're catching the plane back east at eleven or thereabouts."

"Give my regards to the snow," he said.

I said, "I certainly will."

There was another knock on the door. A young man whom I never met introduced himself, and George explained that he was the pharmacist. He handed George a little booklet, containing a description of the medication I would be taking. In the corner of each little page there was, under a stickum wrapper, one pill, so that those of us who could not tell one pill from the other would be able to match it with the medication.

George took the little booklet and handed it to me. "Let's go through this together. Open the first page." I did as he directed. The first page contained information about Digoxin. "Do you remember your medicine, Joe?" he asked.

"A little," I replied. "But let's go through it together as you suggest."

"First, it slows the heartbeat; second, it strengthens the contraction of the heart muscle." George pointed to the little white pill taped on the page. "You're to take one pill a day, preferably after breakfast. Take it the same time every day. If you should forget, take it when you remember, but don't double up on the pill if you should forget it one day. The only side effect you should remember is that nausea or vomiting is to be immediately reported to your doctor. Am I loading you with too much information?"

"Not yet," I replied.

"One other thing. Since you'll be walking, take your pulse before you walk and after you finish. If your pulse is below 58 beats per minute, bring this to the attention of your physician. Then he will adjust your dose as he sees necessary."

"George, will I have to take this for the rest of my life?" I asked.

"I doubt it. That determination will be made by your cardiologist. The next drug is called Coumadin. That's the anticoagulant. You'll need to take this for a while. Since it thins out the blood, you know, reduces the platelet formation so that the blood takes longer to clot, you have to be careful about taking any medication like aspirin. Aspirin seems to have a similar effect and can change your clotting time. You know how fast you clot. This pink tablet of Coumadin you take once a day. Makes no difference what time of the day. By the way, use a soft-bristle toothbrush. Gums tend to bleed easily."

I dislike drugs. I try to use them sparingly in my own practice. Now I was going to be taking a mess of medications. I would take them, but I didn't feel very happy about it.

"George," I interrupted, "You know I'm still having pain in moving my arms, especially my left arm, so what do I take for pain if I can't take aspirin?"

"Darvon," he replied. "You'll find that adequate. It doesn't contain aspirin like many over-the-counter pain killers or so-called remedies for headache. Most of them contain aspirin. Now the last medication I'll want you on is an iron compound. I've prescribed Fergon tablets. Your blood will have to be built up and your hemoglobin levels increased. You won't be on it too long if you eat well. Here again I suggest you follow the directions of your personal physician. He'll be checking your blood picture regularly. He'll be ordering prothrombin to make sure you're not thinning your blood too much, and while doing that, he'll probably check other blood chemistries. Any questions?"

"None at the moment. Let's go over all this once again, can we?"

George repeated all of his directions; I understood and remembered them all. He returned the booklet with the description of the drugs and a sample of the pills taped to each page. I felt exhausted.

"You'll have one more visitor. The nutritionist. She'll give you a list of foods to take and those to avoid. There is a great debate about the connection of diet and coronary artery disease; I prefer that my patients not involve themselves in that clinical debate. But remember that cholesterol is an absolute no-no for you. If anyone tempts you with some nice chocolate, your answer is no."

After all the paperwork was out of the way, George and I began to talk about stress. It was very essential that people who have gone through this heart operation avoid stress. There was no definite correlation between stress and heart disease, but since stress produces certain chemical reactions in a body that produce constriction of the coronary arteries and in turn reduce the amount of blood flow to the muscles, I would have to try to avoid stress.

"Easier said than done," I said.

"Not quite," he answered. "It is necessary that you change your way of life so that these things do not occur. You really must teach yourself to walk away from stressful situations. Avoid them; turn them off; or find some other mechanism that will work. If stress is beginning, let the stress go. Imagine a piece of clay in your hand; that clay is stress. You must learn simply to open your hand and let that clay slip out of the palm and onto the floor. It must not be attached to you.

"The last thing that I have to say to you is the most difficult. You're a physician, Joe. You're accustomed to a patient's recuperating in a few weeks, a month perhaps; then he usually returns to his former routines. But it is not going to be that way with you. Or with any other patient who goes through this. It is going to take more than six months; let me be candid at the moment, and say probably closer to one year. You are really not quite going to feel your oats for about a year. You will have problems climbing the steps. You will feel quite wonderful one day, and then the next find yourself huffing and puffing at the slightest exertion. There is nothing that can be done about this. This is just your body's way of making adjustments. You have a very fine cardiologist and an excellent internist at home. Don't be afraid to see them or call them for any reason at all. Be reassured; it's preferable to experiencing anxiety. Remember, you've got to teach yourself to avoid anxiety.

"And of course," he said, suddenly jovial, with a lilt in his voice, revealing a bit of his Swedish background, "by yumping yimminey, if you don't get any satisfaction from your local M.D. then here is me card and you give me a buzz any time you choose." And he stood up and grasped my hand in a handshake such as I do with my sons. He grabbed me by my thumb and I grabbed him by his thumb and it made the camaraderie absolutely tranquil at that moment. I felt truly sorry to see him leave my room, probably for the last time. As the door was beginning to close, I felt impelled to call out, "Take care, George. I'll miss you." The door silently closed on its hinges, and my words echoed softly in the room, telling me with each echo that I would miss George.

Ten

Eating to Stay Alive

I awoke, hearing my name called. It's only seven in the morning, I thought. It was Carol telling me that the dietician had come to speak to me.

"To both of you," the dietician corrected. She was in her mid-years, wore a white uniform, and carried a stack of papers and two books. She sat beside the bed so that she could face both Carol and me. I wasn't quite sure about this visit. I had a good idea of the kind of diet I was going to have to stay on, but the nutritionist answered a question that I did not even think of.

"I'm glad Mrs. Waxberg is here. Since she's the one who will be doing the cooking, it is important that she understand all the suggestions I'll be making in reference to diet." She had a pleasant voice, and all through our conversation she exhibited great patience with my questions as well as Carol's. "We'll first talk about the subject everyone is interested in, and that is cholesterol. Some doctors do not put much faith in low or absent cholesterol in their patients' food. Here at this hospital, however, we feel it is important to restrict total intake of cholesterol. You know, Doctor, the body manufactures cholesterol regardless of what we eat. On that assumption, we try to diminish even that amount by removing all foods known to contain cholesterol, such as eggs, butter, cheeses, and meat. Some cheeses may be made with skim milk, but you must be very careful to read the labels on all foods you buy. Packaged foods are required by law to list all of the ingredients, and you should make it a habit to read these labels before you buy a product. For example, if the product contains coconut oil, olive oil, or any hydrogenated oil, it would be best to avoid it or find substitutes for that product. Am I going too fast?" she asked.

"Not for me," Carol said.

The nutritionist then continued. "Basically, what we are suggesting is that all foods containing excessive quantities of cholesterol be omitted from your diet. For example, any red meat is going to be filled with animal fat. A nice steak may look and taste good, but the animal fat makes this food dangerous since it is very high in cholesterol. Bacon is another example. A rule of thumb is to eat only poultry — turkey and chicken. Since there is some fat that is mostly in the skin, we suggest you remove the skin before preparing poultry. Cornish hen is acceptable, but remember to remove the skin. Of course, I'm leaving out duck and goose because they are just too high in animal fat; it would be difficult to remove all the fat.

"Perhaps one of the best sources of protein is fish. You can have this fresh, frozen, canned, or even smoked. Fish should be on your diet almost every day as a main course as well as an appetizer. Veal is a source of red meat that is acceptable because the calf is too young to have developed layers of fat.

"I've made out a list of foods, some acceptable and some to avoid. There wouldn't be anough time to go through it all today." She handed Carol several sheets of paper clipped together. I was not too interested in the subject of foods and their proper preparation, but Carol was still reading the sheets of paper intensely after the dietician had left.

"I didn't know that avocado was a no-no," Carol said, still reading the sheets given her.

"So are coconuts and chocolates and cashew nuts and caviar!" I replied.

"Well," Carol said, "from the looks of this list I'm sure you won't starve."

"It's not starving that concerns me," I said. "It really is an entirely new way of thinking about eating. After fifty-five years of one pattern, the need to change is dawning on me. Its importance becomes overwhelming and urgent when you think about it."

"Come to think of it, Joe, how tall are you?" Carol asked.

"The last time I looked, I was about six feet. Right now I feel a foot and a half."

TABLE 1
Ideal Weight for Men and Women
(by frame and in pounds)

	Height	Small Frame	Medium Frame	Large Frame
Men	5'2"	112-120	118-129	126-141
	5'3"	115-123	121-133	129-144
	5'4"	118-126	124-136	132-148
	5'5"	121-129	127-139	135-152
	5'6"	124-133	130-143	138-156
	5'7"	128-137	134-137	142-161
	5'8"	132-141	138-152	147-166
	5'9"	136-145	142-156	151-170
	5'10"	140-150	146-160	155-174
	5'11"	144-154	150-165	159-179
	6'0"	148-158	154-170	164-184
	6'1"	152-162	158-175	168-189
	6'2"	156-167	162-180	173-194
	6'3"	160-171	167-185	178-199
	6'4"	164-175	172-190	182-204
Women	4'10"	92- 98	96-107	104-119
	4'11"	94-101	98-110	106-122
	5'0"	96-104	101-113	109-125
	5'1"	99-107	104-116	112-128
	5'2"	102-110	107-119	115-131
	5'3"	105-113	110-122	118-134
	5'4"	108-116	113-126	121-138
	5'5"	111-119	116-130	125-141
	5'6"	114-123	120-135	129-146
	5'7"	118-127	124-139	133-150
	5'8"	122-131	128-143	137-154
	5'9"	126-135	132-147	141-158
	5'10"	130-140	136-151	145-163
	5'11"	134-144	140-155	149-168
	6'0"	138-148	144-159	153-173

"Here, look at this Joe. This is a table of the weight you should be, depending on your height." The chart we both studied is reproduced as Table 1.

Carol turned to the sheets of paper dealing specifically with the diet. The *amount* eaten, I found, is no less important than *what* is eaten. The information was an eye opener. I could see that my eating habits were going to change radically. There go those potato chip and cookie nibbling late at night! I looked to Carol and it seemed we both had the same thought at the same time. "Goodbye chocolate chip cookies," she said. "And they were so easy to make," I answered. Carol turned her thumb downward.

The full chart is reproduced as Table 2. After reading one page of the list, my eyes became heavy and I fell asleep. It was the *best* way to deal with this superabundance of information at the time.

TABLE 2
Dietary Guidelines

Type of Food	Amount	Foods to Include	Foods to Avoid
Beverage	2 cups milk min.	Skim milk Buttermilk made from skim milk Carbonated beverages Decaffeinated coffee Tea Evaporated skim (1%) milk	Whole milk 2% milk Chocolate drinks and other milk drinks
Meat* Poultry, Fish	8 oz. max. 7 times a week or more	Veal Chicken Turkey Cornish hen	 Poultry injected with butter Poultry skins Goose Duck

*Preparation of meat: Remove all visible fat before preparing. Preferably bake, broil, or roast your meats on a rack so that the fat can drip away. Frying and french frying are permissible if the recommended oils are used.

TABLE 2 (cont.)
Dietary Guidelines

Type of Food	Amount	Foods to Include	Foods to Avoid
		Fish (fresh, frozen, canned, or smoked)	
	To be used less often	Shellfish	
	(No more than 3 times a week)	Lean beef: round steak ground round sirloin tip roast chipped or dried beef arm pot roast cube steak shank flank steak rump roast lean beef stew tenderloin steak porterhouse steak T-bone steak sirloin steak cornered round	Prime grades of beef Other cuts of beef Regular hamburger Frozen packaged convenience foods
		Pork: lean ham loin chops Canadian bacon	All other cuts of pork: sausage, luncheon meats, bacon spareribs, Corned beef Brisket
		Lamb: leg roast loin chops	All other cuts of lamb
		Organ meats: liver. See Eggs 4 oz. once a month	All other organ meats

You may substitute for 3 oz. of meat any of the following:

1 frankfurter or sausage
1 oz. luncheon meat
1 oz. cheese
2/3 cup ice milk

TABLE 2 (cont.)
Dietary Guidelines

Type of Food	Amount	Foods to Include	Foods to Avoid
Eggs		Egg whites Special low cholesterol egg products, such as Egg Beaters	Egg yolks
Cheese		The following cheeses may be used as desired: Baker's cottage cheese Low-fat (1%) cottage cheese Hand cheese — German Gammelost — Norwegian Sapasago — grating Fat-free pot cheese The following may be used if 2 oz. are sub- stituted for 1 oz. of meat: Creamed cottage cheese Regular pot cheese Ricotta cheese Any cheese with a fat content of less than 5% 1 oz. of the following re- places 1 oz. meat: Farmer's cheese St. Otho — Switzerland Any cheese with fat content between 5 and 10%	Any other cheese
Breads and Cereals	4 or more	Any breads: Enriched preferred hard rolls English muffins Bagels Hamburger and hot dog buns Biscuits Muffins Waffles	Cheese bread Egg bread Commercially prepared bis- cuits, muffins,

TABLE 2 (cont.)
Dietary Guidelines

Type of Food	Amount	Foods to Include	Foods to Avoid

		Pancakes
		Baked goods
		Sweet rolls
		Donuts
		Cornbread
		Dinner rolls made
		  with allowed fats
		  and skim milk and
		  allowed eggs
			waffles, pancakes, baked
			goods, etc.

		Plain crackers Saltines Rusk Melba Zwieback Breadsticks Matzoh Graham Rye	Flavored crackers
		Any cereal except ⟶	Any containing coconut
Potatoes		White or sweet potatoes Macaroni Spaghetti Rice Hominy Noodles Baked beans without pork	Potato chips and frozen potato products, unless fried in allowed oil

Vegetables	2 or more	All. 1 dark green or
		  deep yellow daily
		  for Vitamin A
			Vegetables in
			butter or cream
			sauce

Fats	4 tbsp. oil	Oils — in order of preference: Safflower Corn Soybean Sesame seed Cottonseed Sunflower seed	

TABLE 2 (cont.)
Dietary Guidelines

Type of Food	Amount	Foods to Include	Foods to Avoid
		Margarine containing 40% polyunsaturated fat (liquid oil should be listed before the hardened or hydrogenated oil)	Coconut oil Olive oil Peanut oil Butter Margarine high in saturated fat
		Mayonnaise or mayonnaise-type salad dressing	Cream cheese Nondairy cream substitute Cream Half and half Nondairy sour cream Sour cream Nondairy whipped toppings
		Any salad dressing that does not contain sour cream or cheese, such as French, Italian, or Russian	
		Old fashioned *non-hydrogenated* peanut butter	Hydrogenated peanut butter
		Fat-free meat drippings may be thickened with flour; allowed oil or margarine may be added Cream sauce made with skim milk and margarine Imitation bacon bits	Bacon Salt pork
Fruit	2 or more	Any. 1 citrus daily for vitamin C. Avocado only occasionally	
Desserts		Gelatin Fruit ices	Ice cream Ice milk

TABLE 2 (cont.)
Dietary Guidelines

Type of Food	Amount	Foods to Include	Foods to Avoid

		Sherbet
		Meringues
		Any cake, cookie,
		  pastry, or pudding
		  prepared from
		  allowed foods
			Any desserts with
			  foods not al-
			  lowed, such as
			  butter, choco-
			  late, coconut,
			  cream, egg yolk,
			  nuts, whole milk

		Commercial pudding
		  mixes made with
		  skim milk
		Angel food cake
		Frostings made with
		  allowed fat
			Commercially
			  prepared prod-
			  ucts and mixes

Miscellaneous		Nuts. Walnuts preferred,
		  others acceptable,
		  except cashews and
		  macadamia
			Cashews, macada-
			  mia nuts *no*

		Olives occasionally!	

		Most canned or dehy-
		  drated soups except
		  those listed under
		  foods to avoid
		Boullion and fat-free
		  broth
		Homemade soups chilled
		  to remove fat	

		Pretzels
		Home-prepared popcorn
		  made with allowed oil
		Potato chips if fried in
		  allowed oil
			Other deep-fried *no*
			  snacks

		Hard candies ✓ Gum drops ✓ Marshmallows ✓ Honey ✓ Jelly Jam ✓ Chewing gum	

TABLE 2 (cont.)
Dietary Guidelines

Type of Food	Amount	Foods to Include	Foods to Avoid
		Cocoa *yes*	Chocolate *no*
		Salt	
		Spices	
		Herbs	
		Relishes	
		Catsup *no*	
		Mustard *no*	
		Horseradish *no*	
		Soy sauce *no*	
		Worcestershire sauce *no*	
		Texturized vegetable-protein products	

Addendum

The following convenience foods may be used on a low-cholesterol diet

Egg Products:
  Egg Beaters
  Scramble Supreme
  Jolly Joan
  Eggstra

Meats:
  Kelment's roast
  New England ham
  honey loaf

Cheese:
  Fisher's Cheezola
  Fisher's Count Down
  Kraft's Tasty Loaf
  Fisher's Chef's Delight
  Borden's Lite Line

Margarine:
  Chiffon Soft
  Fleischmann Soft
  Mazola Soft
  Nucoa Dream Soft
  Parkay Safflower Soft
  Promise Stick or Soft

Texturized vegetable protein:
  Morningstar Farms sausage, breakfast patties, and ham
  slices

Soup
  Any Campbell's soups *except* cheddar cheese, New England clam chowder, oyster stew, cream of shrimp

The following Campbell's soups should only be used
occasionally:
  Cream of celery
  Cream of chicken
  Cream of mushroom
  Cream of vegetable
  Oxtail
  Pepperpot
  Scotch broth
  Cream of potato
  Snapper

Any Knorr dehydrated soups

Use only the following Heinz soups:
  Beef with vegetable and barley
  Vegetarian vegetable
  Vegetable noodle
  Vegetable beef
  Chicken with rice
  Great American soups

Use only the following Lipton soups:
Tomato
French onion
Beef-vegetable
Chicken with noodles

Eleven

More Instructions for a New Life

I awoke from my nap to find Carol still scrutinizing the information left by the nutritionist. I watched as she read the instructions, page after page.

Just then the door opened and Kathy walked in. She, too, carried a small folder under her arm.

"Apologies from Dr. Shore. He had an emergency this afternoon and he asked me to give you this." She handed me a red cardboard folder containing some papers. "Open the folder, and let's go through them together."

I did as she asked. The first sheet was a schematic drawing of my heart and vessels with the bypasses sketched in. "That's the picture of what was done in surgery. You remember that you were informed about the left anterior descending coronary artery and the blockage that was closing off the vessel. Here," Kathy pointed, "you'll see how the internal mammary artery was used and inserted below the point where the artery was constricted. Now there is no interrupted flow of blood to the heart muscle past that point of blockage. You can also see where Dr. Shore found the beginning of early constriction in the circumflex artery; instead of waiting the ten or twenty years for that vessel to close off and produce symptoms, he decided to bypass that artery as well, as a preventative measure. You'll note that the saphenous vein was used to bypass the circumflex."

I gazed at the drawing trying to absorb what I saw along with what Kathy was explaining. It appeared to be such a simple procedure to correct such a serious, life-threatening condition. (A comprehensive drawing of my bypass surgery is given in Figure 1.)

"Well, here I am, all bypassed and wired together again," I said.

"Any questions about the drawing?" Kathy asked.

"What is the advantage of using the internal mammary artery, Kathy?" I asked. "Many patients I know just had the saphenous vein used. In fact they were never told about the internal mammary artery. I know a little about anatomy and know that this artery travels along both sides of the sternum sending off tributaries to the muscles and bones of the ribcage. But why this artery?"

"The most common reason is that it *is* an artery. Since arteries are anatomically different from veins they'll function almost as well as your own coronary artery. Arteries have muscular walls. They can expand with each pulsation of the heart and take more pressure since they can expand and contract because of the muscle tissue. Now, I'm not saying that veins are not functional. It's just that they are thinner-walled, and although they do an excellent job in the bypass procedure, Dr. Shore prefers to use arteries if he can. In your case it was suitable. The lumen, the diameter, was acceptable, and therefore he used it. Some people's internal mammaries are not sufficiently large to use. In these cases the saphenous vein is placed in position for the bypass. For the small bypass around your circumflex, the vein will serve and survive quite well."

"Have you thought about teaching, Kathy? You explain things so thoroughly and simply," I said. Now I knew why she was such a terrific liaison nurse. I thought how lucky Dr. Shore was to have her.

"Joe had two bypasses," Carol began. "Is there any limit to the number of bypasses a patient can have?"

"I've known of nine bypasses being done," Kathy answered.

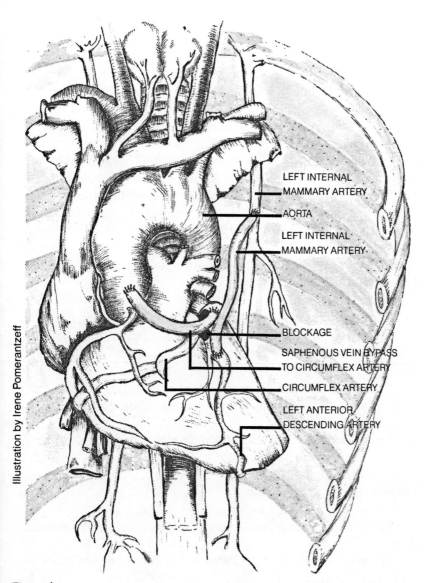

LEFT INTERNAL
MAMMARY ARTERY

AORTA

LEFT INTERNAL
MAMMARY ARTERY

BLOCKAGE

SAPHENOUS VEIN BYPASS
TO CIRCUMFLEX ARTERY

CIRCUMFLEX ARTERY

LEFT ANTERIOR
DESCENDING ARTERY

Illustration by Irene Pomerantzeff

Figure 1

"I notice, Kathy," I said, "that the right side of my heart shows no damage, or at least not now."

"That's right, Doctor. Your right side shows no pathology. Dr. Shore examined every coronary vessel including those in the back part of the heart. No abnormality existed. If there were, then Dr. Shore would have bypassed the vessels in the back of the heart. The result is this drawing that you have before you. It shows exactly what was pathological and what the surgical team repaired. Since there was no other evidence of coronary involvement there was no need for any further surgical intervention."

"Well, that certainly make it clear," I said. "I was wondering how it was done. So Dr. Shore examined the coronary arteries running along the back of my heart. Since he saw no problem with the arteries at the back of the heart, he was able to concentrate on those vessels that were seen as pathological by Dr. Landesman in the angiogram."

"Precisely," Kathy answered. "If the posterior arteries had been involved, we would have seen them on the angiogram, and then Dr. Shore would have visualized them better, once he had your heart exposed. He could palpate each artery and then decide if any of the posterior vessels needed repair."

"That makes sense," I said. "Also so damned simple. I'm sorry I won't be able to say goodbye to Dr. Shore tomorrow before I leave."

Kathy laughed. "I've known him to visit a discharged patient before going to another in surgery. Even if he had to wake up the departing patient. You may be one of the lucky ones; he wakes at five in the morning."

"I wouldn't mind," I replied.

Kathy and I shook hands and I thanked her for all she had done.

"Take care of yourself, Dr. Waxberg." She turned and quietly disappeared through the open door. For a long moment I watched the open door hoping she would return, but I knew there were many other patients she had to see. In a sense I was jealous that I was not the most important. I turned to Carol. "She'll always be someone special to me."

Carol and I walked around the floor, visiting and gossiping

and discussing the advice I'd been getting. Tony was feeling much better; he walked with us.

"The toughest sacrifice I think for me," he said, "is giving up smoking. I even dream about it. I know in one sense it is the worst thing for me and yet I feel it is more relaxing. You tell me, 'Don't be tense,' but what happens to us guys who smoke simply to relax?"

"I wish I had an answer," I said. "I used to smoke, too. I must confess that I'm extremely afraid that once I get home and back into my old routines, I may go back to it again. The next time you fellows meet, try talking about it. Maybe someone may have some ideas or experience he can share."

Even as I spoke, I kept feeling that there was much more to the recovery phase of the bypass operation than had been revealed to me. More important, no one had done much work with the recovery phase. This thought hounded me as we walked and talked. I promised myself that when I got back home I would look into this and probably spend a considerable amount of time in the medical library at Stamford Hospital, studying the post-bypass care of patients.

As we rounded a corner a young nurse approached us. "Dr. Waxberg?" she asked.

"Yes."

"I just stopped by your room and you were gone so I assumed you were out walking. Could we return to your room? I'm the physiotherapist at the hospital and I thought this would be a good opportunity to discuss some of the activities that you should enter into when you return home."

We left Tony. Carol, the nurse, and I returned to the room. On my bed was another folder. She reached for it and handed me the first page. The sheet was entitled 'Discharge Instruction.' I read the first page.

General Activity

Walk: each week increase distance.
First week: ½ mile each day
Second week: 1 mile each day

Third week: 1½ miles each day

Fourth week: 2 miles each day

If cold air bothers you, walk in an enclosed area such as a shopping center or large store. Wear a mask or muffler over nose and mouth if temperature falls below +10°F.

Stairs: Go up and down slowly. Stop and rest if you become tired.

Lifting: DO NOT lift more than 5 pounds until you visit your cardiologist.

Driving: DO NOT drive the first several weeks or until your doctor recommends it. Avoid any strenuous activity such as shoveling snow, mowing grass, or raking in the yard.

Sports: Resume these when your doctor recommends it.

Social activity: Take alcoholic beverages in moderation.

Smoking: NEVER —EVER.

Sexual relations: Discuss with your physician.

Work: Your physician will decide when you can return to work.

Health Care

Weigh yourself every week. If you suddenly gain several pounds, notify your doctor immediately.

Diet: Follow the diet recommended by the nutritionist.

Incision: If it is painful, take pain medication. Bathe or shower as you please. If the incision begins to drain, notify your physician.

Medications: You will receive prescriptions and instructions about the medications you must take when you return home. Please bring the instruction sheet with you when you see any of your doctors.

Exercises

Breathing Exercises: These should be done every 3 to 4 hours during the day and evening.

Arm and shoulder exercises: These should be done several times a day. If you feel stiff in the morning, do these exercises to loosen up.

Isometric exercises: These should be done 5 to 6 times a day so that your chest muscles become strengthened. When you sit, sit erect and don't hold yourself stiff.

"This is most helpful," I said. "I do notice that my left arm, shoulder, and left side of my chest are very stiff and painful. It frequently wakes me, which is most annoying, since I need all the rest and sleep I can get."

"I'm afraid that is going to last for some time," she responded. "Be prepared for at least three months of this type of difficulty. You can help yourself by following these exercises." She handed me the next page from her folder.

Again, I read the instructions.

Home Program

Arm Exercises
1. Arm at side, with elbow straight and palm towards bed. Raise arm up and over head; slowly lower.
2. Arm at side, with elbow straight and palm facing hip. Bring arm out to side and up towards your ear; slowly bring down in circular movement.
3. Bring elbow out to side even with your shoulder, hand pointing up at ceiling. Roll arm backward so that back of hand touches bed; then bend arm forward so that palm touches bed.
4. With elbow at shoulder level, push palms together. Count to 5 out loud (be sure not to hold breath), and relax.
5. Repeat all the exercises above five times each. Increase number of times as stamina improves.

Leg Exercises
1. Bend knee to chest; count to 3, and relax.
2. Tighten buttock muscles; count to 3, and relax.
3. Pull ankles up toward head; push down as far as possible. Be sure to continue practicing deep-breathing exercises twice a day.

When I finished reading the instructions, the physiotherapist handed me the next sheet. "Your chart tells me that you had two bypasses. The stiffness in your shoulder and arms is the result of the work done on the internal mammary artery. It required more surgical time and expertise, but it is more beneficial. I'm sure all this has been explained to you before."

"It has been," I replied.

"However, you still required a saphenous vein removal for the second bypass." Here she stopped to refer to her notes. "Yes, the second bypass was for the circumflex artery. Although in your case the vein was removed from the ankle to just below the knee, you still require as much care as do those patients who have had more of the saphenous removed. Many times the vein is removed from the ankle up to the groin and occasionally both leg veins have to be used. Regardless of the length of the incision, these instructions will be helpful."

Again I began to read, marveling at her patience.

Care of the Leg Incision

At the time of surgery a vein was removed from either one or both of your legs. On occasion, tissues in the lower legs can retain fluid. This is due to an interruption of the lymphatic system, a vessel system that helps to remove tissue fluids. When this system reestablishes itself, the lower leg's tendency to retain fluid should lessen. Meanwhile, you can help minimize any tendency of your legs to swell by elevating your legs in the manner described below.

1. Lie down on either floor, bed, couch, or another flat surface.

2. Elevate your legs higher than your chest by supporting them with a cushion or pillows, or by placing them upon a footstool. Make sure nothing is constricting or pressing against the area behind the knees.

3. Maintain that position with legs elevated higher than your chest for at least 15–20 minutes. Do this three times a day. You may leave the elastic stockings on or remove them when you elevate your legs. You should *remove* the stockings at night.

Your elastic stockings should be worn for approximately two to three weeks after leaving the hospital or until you are able to walk a distance of 2 to 3 miles at one time. Your physician may have you wear them for a longer period of time should your lower legs have a tendency to swell.

If you should travel by car for a long distance, stop every hour to two hours, get out of the car, and walk for 10 minutes or so. By doing so you will help to promote adequate circulation. Should you need to sit for a prolonged period of time, do follow these same guidelines and walk for a while after sitting for one or two hours. Avoid crossing your legs at the knee as this may interfere with good circulation.

Healing of the Incision

Should you be uncertain as to the expected healing process of the leg incision, do not hesitate to call your doctor. It is NOT unusual to detect small spotty amounts of clear, yellow, watery drainage from areas of the incision. If areas of the incision become reddened, warm to the touch, or swollen along the incision, call your doctor. On occasion, skin incisions can become dry and flaky. This condition is only temporary, and nothing is needed to treat it. Keep the incision lines clean by bathing daily, using only soap and water. No lotions or creams are necessary and none should be applied directly to the incision line.

When I finished the page dealing with the leg incision, I said, "This is the most comprehensive day that I've ever had. I have never had an operation in my life except for my tonsils as a kid, but I do want to thank you for your patience and most expert advice. I couldn't help wondering about one last question, however."

"Which one?" she asked.

"The one that refers to sexual activity. How would a family physician be able to answer such a question?"

"I wish I could answer that for you, but I don't think there's been anything published on that question."

"Well," I replied, "as soon as I find out for myself, I may write the first paper.

"I wish you would," she answered. "Interestingly, in all the years I've been doing this work, you are the first to inquire about the question."

"Perhaps the reason is that I'm a sexual therapist as well as a psychiatrist, and when I get back home I may meet with some other patients and find the solution." I thanked her once again, and she left the room, wishing me well and a good recovery.

Carol now had a sheaf of instructions neatly stacked on her lap. "This will be some very interesting reading material for tonight."

"Have fun," I said.

When the nurse brought the dinner tray, I was actually hungry. I asked her whether there was an extra tray around for Carol. I just didn't want Carol to leave early this evening. I had an urgent desire to have her near me and to talk. Tomorrow she would pick me up at 8 A.M. for the plane back to New York, and then we would drive up to Connecticut and home. I sensed apprehension similar to what I'd felt when I'd left the ICU. I wondered whether I would be able to do everything I needed to do without the assistance and help of the staff at St. Mary's Hospital.

After dinner Carol and I walked the floor again. This time I took the Eiffel Tower without fear. I huffed and felt exhausted and could feel my heart pounding, but I felt confident that the new vessels were truly serving their function. Confidence: That's what I was feeling that evening. When we returned to the room, I said, "From now on, Carol, let's celebrate my birthday on December 28, the day of my bypass. I'm one week old today."

"That's a great idea," Carol said. "Christmas and Hannukah and your birthday all rolled into one. Happy one week birthday!"

"How about a kiss to celebrate?" I asked.

"My pleasure."

"Ouch!" I cried. "The pressure of your squeeze hurt! You know, we're going to have to work this thing out some way, but I guess my ardor is greater than my physical capacities."

The remainder of the evening we reviewed some of the material given to us and also the plans for leaving tomorrow. Drowsiness and fatigue began to envelop me slowly and I fell asleep.

I awoke and it was daylight. I'd slept the entire night through. It was 6:30. I could hear dishes being rattled in the hallway: time for breakfast. I showered and shaved. When I put on the suit to travel back home, I had to notch my belt two holes backward. I didn't realize how much weight I had lost. The nurses weighed me in the morning, but I never paid any attention to the figure. I quickly finished breakfast when Carol arrived.

"It's very cold out this morning. About ten degrees."

We finished all the necessary duties such as signing out of the hospital. We said goodbye to all the nurses, and to Tony and Vinnie, who were still sleepy and not quite functioning that early in the morning.

The nurse helped me into a wheelchair, a standard hospital procedure for discharging patients. Carol walked beside us, carrying a suitcase containing all my paraphenalia and what seemed a ton of instructions. She brought the car around and I was wheeled out to the waiting car. *It was cold!* I hopped — better word, *crawled* — quickly into the front seat next to Carol, and off we went.

The wind whipped the snow across the roads making banks in the windward side of every street. Finally, the airport. A porter approached the car and opened the door. Slowly and gingerly I stepped out. "St. Mary's?" he asked.

I couldn't help smiling. "How did you know?"

He helped me inside the warm lobby. "Now don't you move. I'll get a wheel chair." In a moment he was back with the wheels. I thanked him and collapsed into the comfort of the chair. Carol left the baggage with me while she returned the car to the rental agency. As soon as she returned the porter appeared again. "Follow me," he instructed Carol. He wheeled me down the lobby quickly, into an elevator, and then down another lobby. There we stopped before the ticket counter; a stewardess took the wheelchair and steered me to the open door of the jet. Carol followed behind with the baggage. She returned the chair to the porter, helped me walk into the cabin, and seated me on the aisle near the bulkhead where I could have lots of leg room.

"I just don't believe all this," Carol said, strapping herself down and making certain I was comfortable.

"That St. Mary's has some service!" I exclaimed.

As the plane took off and circled over Milwaukee, I looked down, trying to spot the hospital. I couldn't, but, silently, I sent them my deepest thanks and gratitude. Soon the clouds surrounded the plane; I closed my eyes as Carol held my hand.

Twelve

My Friend Ezra

Before we landed at Kennedy Airport the stewardess had called for a wheelchair, but unfortunately none was waiting for me. The temperature was below freezing as we waited for the chair to arrive; I began to feel quite cold and miserable. I couldn't walk too long a distance and we finally entered the massive corridor leading to the exit. I sat on the suitcases waiting for a half hour for the chair to arrive. I was irritable. Carol reminded me about stress, so I resigned myself to waiting. Finally, as Carol and the porter wheeled me to the exit, a wonderful feeling came over me, for warm and affectionate Ron King was waiting patiently for us to appear. His son Peter, who was home from college, accompanied him and we all embraced. I was so thankful for good friends. Peter took the heavy baggage, which Carol had carried so bravely in Milwaukee.

We finally made it to Ron's station wagon. Gratefully, I climbed in and leaned back, happy to be home with friends again. There was a time when I didn't think this day would be a reality. The ride home was slow; I knew Ron was deliberately driving slowly, trying to avoid all the usual hazards of Pothole City. Once we reached the outskirts of New York and headed toward Connecticut, his speed picked up. I don't believe I have ever felt as relaxed and relieved to see our house come in to view as when we drove down the street. It is a beautiful house. It is home and I had made it there. Ron and Peter graciously asked whether there was anything else they could do after the baggage had been brought into the house. I apologized for my weariness; soon I was saying goodbye and thanking them. In five minutes I was luxuriating in my own bed; I stretched once and fell asleep.

When I awoke it was late afternoon. I slowly climbed out of bed and felt the usual stiffness in my left arm and shoulder. I tried to remember the exercises I needed to do. I called Carol and she came into the bedroom carrying all the papers contained in a large folder.

"Do you have the sheet with a description of the exercises?" I asked.

"I just read your mind," she said smiling. In a moment the sheet was before me and I did the arm and shoulder exercise, after which I felt less stiff. I put my bathrobe on, and as I was about to go downstairs I recalled that I'd neglected to put on the white elastic hose. There they were at the foot of my bed.

When I came downstairs I could smell the wonderful fragrance of chicken soup. There was another pleasant surprise standing in the middle of the living room. It was a stationary bicycle.

"Hey!" I called toward the kitchen, "who put this thing here?"

"Ronnie and Peter put it together while you were sleeping." Carol joined me in the living room. "Now, get on and start riding. You need some walking and it's too cold out today. Try pedaling a quarter a mile. There's a speedometer on the machine and an odometer so you can measure how fast and how far you're going."

I swung my leg over and sat on the bicycle and began to pedal. I did a quarter of a mile, but breathing very heavily.

"It's a beginning," I said and I climbed off.

"How about a little chicken soup as a reward?" Carol asked.

"A large bowl."

I devoured the soup. Home cooking, there's nothing like the real thing.

I sat around watching television to distract my mind. It didn't work. I was feeling all sorts of aches and stiffness of joints, and I felt uncomfortable and insecure away from the hospital.

Carol brought the medication I had to take daily. So I swallowed the Coumadin, Fergon, the iron tablet, and the digoxin. I decided that instead of taking them in the morning, I would take them late in the day and established that point of reference for medication time. Usually I found myself uncomfortable, achy and hurting, in the morning and was in no mood for all the medication. As the day wore on, I became more active and more interested and then found the medication acceptable.

That evening Barbara and Bill Ivler arrived. They were good friends of many years. They had returned that morning from the Philippines, where they had been visiting their son, who was attending veterinary school. We talked and chatted about me and about the Philippines; I began to yawn. I apologized, assured them that it was because of fatigue, not boredom. They left and I returned to bed and slept.

I found that I never could sleep the night through completely. If I turned and changed my position, I gasped with the aching of my chest muscles. I would then get out of bed, quietly, so as not to wake Carol, who desperately needed her rest. I would go into the bathroom, open the medicine chest, take one Darvon and return to bed and soon sleep would come.

Visitors arrived; I appreciated their company. Any distraction from myself was welcome. I told no one of my increasing feeling of depression that became a way of life during those first few weeks. I had expected my recovery to come faster. I was anxious to do something—anything. I wanted to go to the office and work. I wanted to exercise. But I was not up to any of this, physically or mentally. I was angry at my own inability to function. Now, not only was I dealing with the depression in secrecy, but irritated at my confinement to the house. Outside, Connecticut was covered with a white blanket of snow. I hated it. It kept me confined to the house. This is the way I existed the first week.

Norman Reader, another good friend, arrived. He is a bank president and it was difficult for him to leave his business, but he did. I remember joking and kidding him for leaving my bank account, as little as it was then, unprotected. He threw a package at me. It contained a jogging outfit: jacket and pants, lined in flannel. I expressed my real appreciation of the gift. We talked awhile. Intuitively, he could tell I was still easily fatigued and he left, admonishing me that I should get outdoors and walk; that would be better exercise than the bicycle machine.

Now it was time for me to see my internist, Don Kanter. Carol had already made the appointment and she drove me to his office. It was good seeing him. His cheerful voice and horsing around with me made me feel immensely comfortable. He examined me from head to toe and then did an EKG. He told me that he saw nothing in it to indicate any pathology. I immediately felt better. A chest x-ray followed. It was most strange for me to see it. There were coils of wires around my sternum.

"That's a lot of wire in me," I said.

"It looks very good," Don answered.

"What are those little white specks over the heart area?" I asked.

"Those are probably metal clips that Dr. Shore used to clamp off small blood vessels."

I didn't like all that metal in me. I admitted I didn't understand it. "Why not use plain sutures?" I asked.

"I'm no surgeon," Don replied, "but if Shore used clips, that's his technique, and I'm sure that's the best decision. Clips are so much easier and faster to apply than sutures. Perhaps sutures can loosen or slip off. I don't know. But I suspect whatever Shore did was the correct and responsible thing to do."

Then Don took some blood to test for my clotting time since I was still on the blood-thinning medication. I learned that I needed weekly tests to make certain that the Coumadin was doing its job and that I was not taking too much or too little.

After the examination Don told me that everything looked fine. I was still not quite convinced, and I was concerned about the muscle chest pain. "Suppose it's angina and I confuse it with muscle soreness?" I asked.

"Do you have that feeling now?" Don asked.

"Constantly," I replied.

"Well, it's not angina. If it were it would show in your EKG, but the EKG is normal. You know, Joe, it's a strange thing to say, but at least you know what you have in your chest. You know what your heart is like. The coronaries that were constricted have been bypassed. I repeat, you at least know what you have. I don't. I have no idea what's in my coronaries; that is, unless I have an angiogram myself. At least you were a good enough physician to recognize the first attack of angina on your own and go to the hospital that night. I often think about those patients who know something is wrong and yet do nothing about it. Then they die. Is it the fault of the physician? No, I think we have to really educate the public to recognize these symptoms and have them checked out immediately. I'm not saying you're lucky. What I'm saying is you're smart. Intelligent enough to have acted on those first symptoms, without waiting."

"I suppose you're right," I said. I remembered some of my friends who had died suddenly. That left anterior descending coronary artery was the culprit proven after autopsy. I, at least, was still walking around.

Don closed his folder and made another appointment to see me.

The weather was getting slightly better toward the middle of January. Although it was still very cold, I would bundle up first in the jogging outfit Norman Reader had given me, adding two warm, heavy ski sweaters, a woolen scarf around my throat, and a sheepskin coat on top of all that. I also wore fur-lined gloves and a large woolen hat. Then I would walk. There was a flat piece of road that ran along a lake used as a reservoir. I liked the smell of the pine trees ringing the lake, and the little traffic did not bother me. I would walk slowly, trying to pace myself, each day increasing the time I walked. Soon I was walking three miles a day at a rather brisk pace. But I still was weary.

At least once a week my depression would be very severe and incapacitating. I was expecting too much of myself, and there was no one around with whom I could compare notes about my feelings. I found myself anxious and calling Richard Landesman, my cardiologist, for appointments. An EKG would be done; he would reassure me and then gently urge me to continue with the exercises. Usually, in a week I would be back in his office. A new feeling in my chest would make me anxious; in reality, it was just a sign of the normal healing process taking effect. His patience was beyond anyone's I knew. The same routine. He would listen to my chest and take another EKG. In retrospect I felt his presence and reassurance was a vital part of my recovery.

After Vinnie had been discharged, he and I, like two blind mice, would compare symptoms, not knowing what they meant. It was time to do something about all this, I thought.

Meanwhile I kept working at the exercises, building up my stamina. I began to notice that after a workout I felt more elated, more confident in myself, and I understood the constantly changing symptoms in my chest. I began to lift about five pounds in the morning with each hand to loosen the stiffness in my joints. Each day I'd lift the five pounds and just bend my elbow with the weight, and then lift my arms above me. It made movement easier the remainder of the day. Evening hours of sleep still were not consistent. I would toss and turn, awake with the pain in my shoulder and left arm; a Darvon would help, and I would be able to return to sleep.

When I saw Vinnie, he had new symptoms, such as severe numbness of his left forearm down to his little finger and ring finger. I suspected it was from the stretching of the brachial plexus, the nerves supplying impulses to his left arm down to his finger tips. But I wasn't sure, and he hesitated to ask his physician. However, his symptoms vanished inside of a matter of months.

I began meeting other physicians and patients who had had bypass surgery and soon found myself suggesting that we meet at my house or theirs or during our walks to compare some of our experiences. Still, none of us had explanations that fit all symptoms.

One evening Monroe Coleman and his wife Elaine arrived. Monty and I played golf often and I knew he had severe angina, especially when climbing the hills on the golf course. I would wait for his angina to diminish and then slowly we would walk up the hill. Now that I had had the bypass, he seemed interested in the whats, wheres, and whys of my surgery.

"Thinking of having one?" I asked.

"One never knows," he answered.

"Never to allergists," I replied. "With all the running around to give those shots it would seem you get sufficient exercise. Psychiatrists tend to sit on their butts all day." Elaine wanted our conversation discontinued and I didn't blame her.

"Let's walk through the house, Joe," she suggested. She took my elbow and slowly guided me from one room to the other, maintaining a pleasant running conversation and accomplishing two things: first, walking me around, and, second, ending the topic of medicine.

After our walk we had some tea; they had cake and I had a small slice of toast and jam. Oh, well, I thought, this is going to become a way of life. But that was the first time I was aware of my new eating patterns, since we had had no one over for dinner yet and I was not yet interested in or capable of going out to dine. I remembered looking at the chocolate cake. I found myself interested in my own action. The cake was a threat to me, as if taking a slice of cake would immediately clog my coronaries. It took almost a year to rid myself of the fear of going off my diet. If I was going to follow instructions, I was going to do exactly that, without any deviation. At least those were my convictions that evening.

Days passed with the same routine, the sameness of one day following the next, except for the occasional panic of a chest pain that would be reassured by Dick Landesman. I'd get off his examining table feeling foolish as hell but also feeling better, for now the panic had subsided. I wondered whether other patients had this same problem. Vinnie told me one day he agreed with me, but he thought he would be embarrassed if he ran to his cardiologist and it turned out to be nothing.

"But suppose it *was* something?" I asked. "Something serious?" He shrugged his shoulders and we continued our walk in silence. There had to be some sort of guidance. After I left Vinnie, I was still pondering the question when I noticed another man approaching me at a very fast pace. He was walking, not jogging. As he drew near, I called out, "Bypass?" He stopped and with a smile he turned and crossed the road to my side.

"You, too?" he asked. I nodded and introduced myself; we shook hands, both wearing heavy gloves, and began to walk together. I learned he was in advertising; he was fifty-nine; and he lived a mile from where we met, with his wife and two college-aged daughters. His surgery had been performed three months ago at a New York City hospital. We chatted and continued to walk.

Now here he was, George, by name, operated on at a different hospital, by a different internist and cardiologist. But we had one thing in common, the bypass. He also told me that his operation was performed three months ago, and that he had had three bypasses done.

Near the bend in the road I had parked my car. I invited him to my house to continue our bull session and planned to drive him home after our talk.

George was interested in the schematic drawing I had been given in Milwaukee.

"This is great," he said. "I wish they had done something like this for me. What's an internal mammary?"

I tried to explain about the internal mammary artery and the whys and wherefores of its use. Only saphenous veins had been used by his surgeon. I would have felt uneasy if he had questioned me about its use, but he didn't. I couldn't answer and simply said that each surgeon uses different techniques. George had had angina before surgery but it was now gone.

I invited George to have lunch with me. We had a salmon salad, a slice of toast with margarine, and a glass of skim milk. We talked some more during and after lunch, promising to meet again. George called his wife, who picked him up, saving me the trip. We both understood it was time for a nap for the two of us.

I kept meeting other former patients on my walks along the reservoir or at the YMCA. Slowly I had congregated about six patients including myself. We would meet at various homes to have rap sessions.

I still had weekly visits with Don Kanter. My prothrombin time had to be watched. He was most encouraging, always admonishing me to exercise. Occasionally I would want to know how long this recovery phase would last. It was difficult for me to cope with my physical exhaustion. I knew he couldn't answer my question, but who could?

I pondered the question repeatedly. Then I had the most obvious answer right before me. My friend, Ezra Epstein, the

physician who was my internist before he himself had had a bypass. Unfortunately, his bypass had had some rather severe complications, and as a result he was unable to practice. I knew he
was in Florida for the winter, on Sanibel Island, and he had sent
some flowers to me at St. Mary's. I found the answer. Ezra, my
old friend of over twenty years' duration. He was more than a
friend, he was an excellent internist. He is that rare type of
physician in whom I trusted and believed. The paranoid reaction that I found myself occasionally going through while I was
at home after surgery began gnawing away at me; I found myself thinking that I must be with Ezra because Ezra would tell
me the truth. I wanted to speak to him, to see him, to watch
his face as we discussed my bypass and his. In other words, I
wanted to compare operations and I wanted to know whether
or not what I was feeling was what I *should be* feeling. Or if
what I was feeling was what I should *not* be feeling.

Connecticut, that particular January, was hounded and har-
ried by polar winds, ice and snow, and other afflictions. I
thought of the ten plagues visited on the Egyptians by Moses,
although I had doubts that any plague that took place in Egypt
was happening in less than 80 degree temperatures. The plague
of ice and snow prevented me from exercising, which was essential to my recovery. Walking, to be exact, was supposed to be my
number one exercise. It was my first act of returning to the living.
At least I was repeatedly told by all the physicians that I had to
walk. Those internists and cardiologists who were my dear
friends and still are, Donald and Richard, performed their
Dracula-like feats of drawing blood for prothrombin time. They
had to know if I was clotting too fast, and making small thrombi
skittle up my legs and to see whether my iron content was adequate. Finally, the word arrived that I was well enough to
travel, so off I went to Sanibel Island to be checked by the real
expert, my friend Ezra — the one who had gone this road years
before and knew every inch of the way; he could guide me.

When we first met, I waited and wished for his words; like a
disciple to guru, I sat at his feet. Would I live? Recover? Was I
doomed to invalidism? But it didn't happen that way. I could
lie and write that heroic lines were exchanged between us, but
the truth was less dramatic.

When we'd driven from the airport and settled in the apartment that we had obtained, there was a note on the door from Roz and Ez inviting us to please come directly to their apartment for dinner as soon as we were settled. Carol and I did exactly that, because she knew my reason for coming to this strange island of Sanibel.

Before we walked into their apartment, which was on the second floor, I recall walking up the steps and wondering if I would make it. I felt there were at least a thousand steps to climb; each step seemed to drain my energy, of which I had so little left. When we got to the top, I did not allow Carol to knock on the door, nor would I, until a few minutes had passed, permitting me to catch my breath. I would not have Roz and Ez see me gasping for air like a hooked fish.

Finally, when I was breathing normally again, I knocked on the door. Ezra opened the door and he said, "Damn it, you look great. A little pale, perhaps, but one day in the sun and tomorrow you'll be tan!"

Then Roz came over. She gave me a kiss and we exchanged the usual greetings. I remember that I then said to Ezra, "You look positively fantastic. How are you feeling?"

Ezra, taking one of those mock poses of pumping iron and flexing his muscles like Arnold Schwartznegger, said "I feel great."

Roz added, "Ezra has begun jogging."

Looking at him, I said to myself, "It is three years since he was operated on. It is true his was a very difficult recovery. He had developed pericarditis, which was very difficult for him to overcome. This very severe infection in the lining of his heart took so long to resolve that he had had to give up practice completely, because he could not maintain any activity. He retired from medicine, which was a great loss. My first impulse was to ask, 'Is this going to happen to me, too?' But I did not say it. There are times when it's best not to verbalize one's thoughts."

"You're just in time for dinner," he said. "I've been cooking chicken without its skin, so you will have no fat."

"How thoughtful," I replied. "Without any fat. I hope I'm not putting you out."

"And then we're going to have a little celebration because we

have a special dessert." He talked on and on about food, but I
had no appetite. I wanted just to sit on the couch with him so
that I could bombard him with my questions and he could relieve me of my anxiety. But I was not to have my wish granted
at that particular moment.

Roz and Carol kept up a steady flow of conversation. They
had something new in common now: each was married to a
physician who had had coronary bypasses. I imagined, even
though I could not hear their conversation, how they would go
through the entire operation together: "And then he did this,
and then he did that, and he treated me this way, and treated me
that way." "Oh, you poor dear, I know how you feel." But I am
sure, too, I am over-dramatizing that particular point. I am sure
they said none of these things.

At dinner we gossiped about Stamford and other physicians:
who was doing what to whom; whose practice was doing well
and whose practice was doing poorly; who was taking in new
associates; who was not taking in new associates — all that *crap.*
I said to myself, "Oh, guru, why don't we cut out this small
talk and let me ask these questions! I am getting so choked up
that your marvelous charcoal-grilled chicken with the skin removed is making me gag." I tried to swallow the food, but I
left most of it on the plate. Roz asked whether I was feeling
well, because I did not finish. I lied to her, saying that I had had
a large meal aboard the plane and was not really hungry. I was
most eager for dinner to be over so that I could turn the conversation and manipulate the subject matter to what I wanted it to
be. But it was a difficult task to do anyway, and ultimately dinner did end. It seemed as though hours had passed and I was
feeling rather fatigued. I suspect that my fatigue was mostly
the result of the tension and anxiety I had been experiencing
throughout the meal.

We finally walked into the living room and I was still having
some problems, because after eating, my thoughts do go to my
pipe and smoking. Ezra seemed almost to read my mind and
offered me some gum, handing me a pack of sugarless gum,
such as I had been consuming in tremendous quantities since I
had surrendered my pipe. I imagine that the amount of gum I
chewed could have made a ball the size of the Unisphere at the

New York World's Fair. I chewed, waiting for Ezra to get settled. Although I didn't want to rush the conversation, I found
myself again making attempts to manipulate the subject most
important to me, but each time I began, one of our wives or
Ezra would make some comment about the family or some
other nonmedical topic.

After two minutes, it seemed that hours had passed in idle
conversation, and I could not bear postponement of the inevi-
table any longer; I turned to Ezra and said, "My left arm is kil-
ling me. Is this a common occurrence after surgery?"

He laughed. "Yes, Joe, it's a common occurrence, and you
might as well resign yourself to it because your muscles and
your bones have to heal. It's going to last six months to a year,
and sometimes it's going to be very painful."

I reached for another stick of gum with my right hand and
felt a severe pain in my ribs; for the first time since my operation, I could put up with it. I massaged the area until the pain
left. For the first time, too, I had no anxiety about the pain.
This is not angina after all, I told myself; Ezra said this is a common occurrence.

I tried to act nonchalant and blasé about the whole matter. "Really?" was my only response. Then came question two:
"You know, I've wondered how long it takes for the incision on
the sternum to heal."

"Let's take a look at it," he said. I lifted up my polo shirt
and let him examine my suture line.

Roz said, "That looks marvelous, Joe."

Ezra added, "That is fantastic. Did you have a plastic surgeon do this?"

"Plastic surgeon?" I asked.

"Oh, yes," he explained, "my daughter-in-law's father had a
bypass, and while he was in the hospital—she's a nurse, you
know—requested that a plastic surgeon come by and do the
suture line after the operation."

"How vain," I thought to myself. "A plastic surgeon? I was
so glad to get the damn operation over with, to find that my
eyes could open and I could breathe and move around. A plastic
surgeon indeed!"

"No, there was no plastic surgeon."

"It is marvelous," he said.

He lifted his own polo shirt, so that I could see his scar. I was a little embarrassed. "Ezra, that's a keloid formation," I said. A keloid formation is a type of scar tissue that has healed very thickly and has raised from the skin. It doesn't heal with a nice smooth surface that ultimately is absorbed and covered over by the new skin, but forms a thick elevated scar. And he ran his finger down his scar, saying, "Yes, it is a keloid formation. What can I do about it? That's the way I heal. I heal with keloids. But, Joe, yours is great. In a year you won't even notice it."

I began to feel better, but did not want to give him the impression that I was overwhelmed with the fact that my scar was going to heal differently from his. I tried to sound sarcastic: "Thanks for the compliment, but I still feel lousy."

Reaching for the third piece of gum, I asked, "How does one know if one has angina? I've never had angina. I had this sort of discomfort which I interpreted as indigestion. How do I know if I really have angina?" And Ezra looked at me again, and the tone of his voice changed, as if I were some child that he was trying to lecture. A child with a very low IQ. Frankly, he made me feel retarded and he explained that if one has angina, one does not forget the pain as it is very painful, cruelly so, terrifyingly so, and I said again, "How would I know when to recognize it, because the pain in my chest, as it's healing, is painful."

"Ah," he answered, "but it is fairly constant." And I admitted that.

He said, "Angina is very different, Joe. I'm not going to go into details about it, though, because I am concerned that you'll start looking for it and imagining you have it." For a moment I was angry at his condescension, but I knew he was quite correct and I knew he knew me, and I loved him for the manner in which he was treating me this evening.

I couldn't stand being put off any longer. "Ezra," I said, "you know, I'm absolutely terrified. I don't know what to expect. I don't know what things I feel. I don't understand what I feel. I don't know what it means. It worries me that I'm misinterpreting what I feel. It's driving me up a tree."

Ezra's tan facial appearance changed. His voice, usually, has a nice timbre, gentle and firm, with a little bit of a twinkle. He loves puns and jokes, but this time his voice changed and he suddenly became very professional and not a friend, but a physician. "What are the medications you're taking now, Joe?" I told him I was taking one Coumadin to keep my blood from clotting, because apparently I needed it for the vein that they had removed from my right leg. He interrupted me by saying, "You don't have to explain the reason you're taking the medication, Joe, I'm quite aware of it."

Once again I felt like a small retarded child, and I then continued, "I am taking Digoxin, and iron tablets — I guess I may be anemic — and a multiple vitamin. For the pain in my arm and shoulder, I take some Darvon, and when I get very anxious, I take a Valium."

"One Valium," Ezra asked, "or two or three, perhaps."

I admitted "I sometimes took more than one."

"What exercises were you told to do?"

And I explained that I had to walk at least a mile a day, and increase the distance to two or even more if I could, and I had to perform my arm-raising exercises described to me back in Milwaukee — up and to the sides. I had been told not to jog and not to push myself, but that it was very essential that I do the walking.

And he said, "Fine. Tomorrow you can start, although the weather has not been quite good. It is cold, and the temperature in the morning is between 40 and 50 degrees."

"I don't care." I replied. "as long as there's no snow. I'll just bundle and walk as much as I can."

"Fine," he said again. "And when you get tired and you come by, I'll be sitting out on the beach in back of the house here; we'll chat after your walk."

"Sounds great," I said.

He looked at his watch, and said, "It's almost ten. "Why don't you and Carol go back and get some sleep now, and we'll see you tomorrow."

As a matter of fact, right then I yawned in his face, so we called it a day.

Thirteen

A Moment of Holy Reassurance

Carol and I settled in for our first night at Sanibel. The day had passed quickly. The dinner and the visit all seemed to fly — the sun passed the horizon. In the dark we walked back to our apartment.

"That talk I had with Ezra did me a world of good," I said to Carol.

"I've noticed. Your face is more relaxed, and your posture is straighter when you walk, and more assured."

I took out a pad that I had brought with me and began making entries of our talks. These notes were to be the beginning of a paper that I wanted to publish about my experiences. I wrote that the pain and cramping were to be expected and that patients should not overemphasize the disagreeable aspects of the healing process. We had to be patient; body changes were going to last from six months to a year; and for some patients, healing would take even longer.

Being Type A individuals, we all would have to overcome the competitiveness among ourselves when the group began to meet with some regularity.

I reexamined my notes, adding other thoughts that had

come out of my conversation with Ezra. Although he seemed
extremely well adjusted, I knew him to be a Type A personality
from years back. I pondered about the appeal of medicine to
those students who were of this nature.

I awoke the following morning anxious to have breakfast.
I was starved, a condition I had not experienced for over a
month. I had bran flakes with a sliced banana, orange juice, a
slice of toast, margarine, and a cup of coffee. I put on Norman
Reader's jogging outfit, and since the temperature was still in
the upper forties, I wore my sheepskin coat on top of my
jogging outfit.

I stepped out onto the beautiful white beach. It was now
7:30 in the morning. The seagulls accompanied me as I paced
myself northwards, into the wind. I walked to the edge of
Sanibel, then turned and headed south. I walked more than five
miles that morning. I felt energetic, and happy about my guru,
Ezra. As I approached his house, he was sitting in the sun,
reading the newspaper; Roz was beside him, feeding him raisins.
Carol was already there when I joined them. I collapsed on a
beach chair and felt for my pulse.

"What are you doing?" Ezra asked.

"What does it look like? I'm trying to see whether I've
reached about 140 beats per minute."

"Look, Joe," Ezra began, "This is not the place to count
pulses. Relax. Enjoy the sun and our company,"

"I guess you're right, Too much Type A?" I asked.

"No, too much apprehension. I wish they never coined
that damn term, *Type A*. Some people are tense and anxious all
day, that's all. They do not know how to relax, have to have
booze and constant distractions like people, or television or
arguments or you name it, as long as it keeps them from thinking of themselves. You one of them?"

"That's me! I had coronary artery disease, so I suppose I'm
Type A."

"Such baloney!" Ezra exclaimed. "Genetics is the answer,
Joe. Think about your own family. Your father died young;
uncles and a few aunts died young. You come from a cruddy
genetic background. Start there. Forget Type A."

"Thanks for your encouragement. If I'm to believe what you're saying, there is no way that I could have prevented what happened to me."

"That's right," Ezra said.

"It seems the odds are against anyone with a history that, genetically, is similar to mine or yours."

"Now you're learning." He popped a few more raisins in his mouth. "If there were some way we could pick our antecedents, our predecessors, we'd be in great shape. But then if we could, I don't think this world would be the same. Who knows? I dislike the idea of picking a nucleus from an ovum for only one reason without really understanding what that might do to the rest of the body. This business of cloning is a very frightening concept for humans. Fine for animals, but just fraught with problems for the thinking human."

"I feel the same," I replied. "There are psychiatrists who choose the most casual comments about schizophrenia — suggest that the disease is transmitted genetically. If we tried to fix it, I would worry that we would shake up some other part of that chromosome. A monster, a passive patient, no aggressivity — I don't know. Something would be different. You simply cannot tamper too much with Mother Nature. She had a few billion years to develop our species. I think I'll just go along with her for awhile. Mice and rats are one thing. Humans, well, I'm not too sure."

We arose together, each deep in his own thoughts, and we walked slowly up the beach. As we walked I picked up some interesting shells and put them in a small plastic bag I carried. The shells were too beautiful to ignore, and Sanibel is truly the shell picker's island.

After a period of silence, I felt it was time to ask a question that had begun to distress me lately.

"Ez, when is it safe to have intercourse? I've been feeling — well, you know, a bit horny, but I've been fearful."

"A fellow named Stein, who teaches at Downstate Medical School in New York, wrote a paper about this," Ezra said. "But the paper dealt with those patients who had had myocardial infarcts — neither one of us has had a heart attack — but he did say that if one can climb a flight of stairs, one can have sex. The amount of energy needed for intercourse is less than that for the simple task of climbing stairs."

"I think I'm ready," I said.

Ezra laughed and joked about my testosterone levels being sky high. "Who knows?" I asked.

"Who cares!" he replied. "It's one of those questions that each patient must answer for himself."

We returned to his part of the beach. Roz had already prepared a lunch of salad and tuna fish, which I devoured while sitting in the sun. My anxiety had diminished considerably. We talked the rest of the afternoon about our families and our children and made the usual gossip. I felt energetic and I wanted to walk again. Although Ezra declined to join me, I stretched my legs and off I went, doing four miles that afternoon. The sun was setting at about six and we decided to go out for dinner. We picked a nice seafood restaurant and ate fish, more salad, and bread. We refused the butter and informed the waiter to suggest to the chef he put in a supply of margarine. It went completely over his head. How can one want a substitute for butter?

We returned about nine and I was very tired. I had done a great deal of walking that day. Because of my talks with Ezra, I had more energy and more stamina. He made me feel at ease, and for the first time I was taking my recovery phase in stride. Everything was going well. I loved the time I spent with Ezra. I do not know how any patient can get through the period of recuperation without assurance from someone who had gone through a similar operation. The multitude of questions and doubts and the many other aspects of recovery become much easier to understand when there's someone to discuss them with.

Back in my own apartment, I undressed and watched a little television. When I found my eyes slowly fighting to stay open, I announced, "I think it's time to hit the sack."

"That's fine with me," Carol answered. "I think I got a little sunburn sitting in the sun."

"You look beautiful" I said. "The tan becomes you."

We went to bed and in a moment I was asleep.

When I awoke, I was wide awake. My eyelids refused to

close, as though they had been mysteriously touched with some glue that would prevent them from ever closing again. Every time I would close my eyes in the attempt to return to sleep, my thoughts would make them pop open again like a jack-in-the-box. I stared ahead of me and saw only darkness.

I rolled over on my back, which was a more comfortable position. The pressure against my breast bone was lessened, allowing me to take deep breaths without any difficulty, and the muscles in my chest were not continuously reminding me of the steel sutures that held the sternum together.

I could hear the grandfather's clock in the livingroom, going tick, tock, tick, tock. Carol's steady breathing reassured me that the house was in perfect order. That is, everything was working the way it should, except for me. At three in the morning, I should have been asleep.

I knew, too, that I had exercised much of the day. I could get up, I told myself, go to the medicine cabinet, and take another Dalmane or a Darvon; that would diminish the muscle pain which, perhaps, was keeping me awake. But I didn't want to get up out of bed. I liked hearing the sounds of the apartment; they were comforting. I rolled onto my side so that my body contoured against Carol's body, like two matching pieces of a jigsaw puzzle. With one hand that I placed gently around her stomach, I could feel her even breathing, my hand being lifted and lowered with each gentle breath. For the first time in weeks I felt a stirring in my loins that was like a miracle to me. I had thought about this moment countless times, always privately, quickly hiding the thought or pushing it from my mind. I doubted that I would ever be aroused again, but here it was. I recalled Ezra's remark about climbing stairs.

My desire to wake Carol was selfish, I felt. She had to be exhausted from running around, doing the millions of little things that I required or requested so that I would be spared overexertion. I cradled her in my arms and held her close, and smelled the back of her neck. And it was *her* smell.

I recalled my son once asking me how a sheep knew which lamb belonged to her. I explained that each sheep recognized its own lamb by smell; each has a distinctive odor. He thought I was kidding, because all sheep smelled the same to him. As I smelled the woman I loved, I recognized her truly. Hers could be blended and mixed and distorted with thousands of other odors, and, I guarantee you I would be able to pick it out, 100 times out of 100 tries.

I softly kissed the back of her neck, and held her closer. Then I knew she was awake. It was the most subtle form of communication between two people. Her body, which was next to mine, was aware. The gentlest movement of her hips against my groin — so gentle, hardly measurable, yet I could recognize it. And again, that signal from her body against mine, and from my body against hers. My stirrings now became feelings of strength and power that I did not think I would ever have again; they seemed to be welling out of my groin. I craved to make love to her. I maneuvered my body so that I could fulfill this desire. My chest ached and I had to wait a moment — a moment of eternity — until the pain and discomfort left me. My desire was heightened by her response to me; it was as important to her to be around me as to have me inside her. For the first time since the surgeon's knife had penetrated me, I felt alive; I felt capable of living again.

It was a mystical moment. It was a holy moment that finally came, a moment of reassurance and I felt that my phoenix had arisen from the fire.

I couldn't ignore the pain accompanying every movement; moreover, each time I reached for her, the physical memories and reactions impinged themselves, and I had to fight that part of my brain that sent messages of pain from my muscles, distracting me from the tenderness I wanted to express. I fought. I was determined not to relinquish my sexual excitement to anything. Had my sternum torn open and my lungs eviscerated at the moment that I penetrated, I would not have been stopped.

I entered from the rear in the side position. Her body welcomed me, and I was alive. My heart pumped and the new vessels pumped; the moment of climax came rapidly because it had been such a long time. In my ears I could feel my pulse pounding loudly, but I was alive. I shouted to myself. I was alive!

In the darkness, neither of us moved. I remained in her,

attached to her, not wanting to separate. Forever, I said to myself, forever to feel this way. To be this way.

My chest heaved, and I gasped for air, but I did not care. Had that been the last memory of my life, it would have been worth it. That it was not the last moment of my life was a delightful surprise, I thought. Soon my breathing was restored and the room was quiet again, and my loved one very softly whispered, "That was nice." And I was very happy. I held her close, and as each moment ticked away, I could feel the strength of my arms around her ebbing; so that my grip was loosening, centimeter by centimeter, and my tumescence was slowly ebbing like the gentlest of all tides. I smelled her again. The texture of her skin and moistness of our bodies that were locked together — these were the last things I was aware of that night.

Now I was not afraid to close my eyes since I knew I was going to *be* alive and I *was* alive, that I would *remain* alive. And for the smallest, plainest fraction of a moment, a thought whisked into my mind, "Could I do it again?" My ears heard the question and my intercostal muscles gave me a twitch, simply to remind me they still were there. And all these events happened with such rapidity that as I closed my lids the last thought was, again, — I am alive! I opened my mouth and kissed the back of her neck. "I love you," I said. I slid into a beautiful, restful sleep, such as I had not had for many, many weeks.

That morning I sang in the shower while Carol was making breakfast. I became breathless after soaping one half of my body. I had to sit down on the edge of the tub and wait till I'd caught my breath. But I did not worry about it, and I did not feel anxiety. When I caught my breath again, I continued to soap the other half of the body and slowly rinsed it off. While I dried myself, I went through the same process — when I got tired, I just stopped and then continued the drying process until it was all completed, and put on my jogging suit in which I was going to walk. I had breakfast — orange juice, one Digoxin tablet, one Coumadin tablet, one iron tablet, one vitamin tablet, bran flakes with a sliced banana, and a small piece of toast with margarine. I was happy that I was with Ezra and felt safe.

Carol dressed quickly and we went walking out towards the

beach. The beach was beautiful and white, glistening in the sunlight. There were three lines of shells—one very far up the beach, probably left by high tide; one sort of midway, probably left by the last tide; and one very close to the edge of the water. We walked northward at first, into the wind, because I had more energy when I first started to walk. I wore a heavy ski sweater that protected me from the wind (the weather was in the high fifties). I don't know how far we walked, but we walked at least 15 to 20 minutes going out and another 15 to 20 minutes going back to Ezra's apartment, where he and Roz were sitting again in the sun. We joined them.

"How is the psychiatrist this morning?"

"Pretty good, Ezra," I said. "Much less anxiety and a little stronger."

He said, "I never understood how you, who have spent so many years on a couch learning all about yourself, could feel anxiety. You're a great disappointment to me, Joe."

I felt defensive and said to him, "This is no ordinary panic attack, Doctor, and this is not anything unreal, Doctor. This is quite real and something that almost killed me. How did you expect me to act, like someone without feelings and emotions?"

He dimissed me with a wave of his hand. "All you psychiatrists are just neurotics."

I smiled at him. "Yes, Ezra, whatever you say." Dropping my facetious tone, I thanked him for his comments the night before. "You relieved me of much of my anxiety. All my questions, stupid as they were, you answered. And that made me feel good."

For a moment he simply looked at me. Ezra is not a very touching type of person, and not sentimental, at least in my memory, and his hand came across a twenty-year gap. He grabbed my wrist and held it, and he said to me, "How fortunate that you have no complications, Joe, that you did not have to go through what I had to go through! How fortunate that you are nothing but a dumb shit psychiatrist instead of an internist who knows so much more about cardiology. I recall the days I would lie in bed myself, analyzing and thinking, and being terrified by all the things I knew. The truth of the matter is, Joe, I knew too much and that sometimes is not a very good thing." He patted my arm again. "Feel like taking another walk?" I looked up and I smiled at him. I wanted to hug him actually, but I said to him, "Yes, I would like to take a walk," and we stood up. We walked southward on the beach, with the wind.

Fourteen

The First Stress Test

The next few days I was filled with an energy that I did not feel prior to my visit with Ezra.

Each morning I would walk along the beach as fast as I could. A jogger I met pointed out two landmarks that equaled the distance of one mile. I would warm up by slowly walking to this landmark and then increase the pace for the measured mile. I clocked the time. The first walk, I did the mile in twenty-two minutes. Each morning I would try again to walk faster, but I wasn't able to break that time. Feeling energetic, I would begin by walking very briskly, until I was breathing very heavily and had to slow down until my breathing returned to normal, I would repeat the process. I tried to do at least two miles a day, and occasionally three. I also began to walk in the afternoon trying to do at least another mile. Afterwards, we would all meet at Ezra's apartment and continue bantering about the philosophy of medicine, particularly about the effects of the bypass on the recovering patient.

One morning, as Ezra and I were walking, he said, "You astound me, Joe. You're walking at a great pace and your dedication is encouraging. How are the symptoms?"

"I still have them. I often awake at least once in the evening and have to take a Darvon or a Dalmane to get back to sleep. But I seem to have lost all the anxiety and excessive concern about the symptoms. I know I'll have the symptoms. You explained that recovery will take quite a while. I've also noticed that my obsession with my own mortality has diminished. I know we're all going to die, but I don't think I'd like to know my own time beforehand. Do you understand? It's like — well, all right, I had the operation and I'm glad it's over. I also know it was a life saver; that is, in time that coronary vessel would have closed off completely and, gafooey — all over. This second chance made me shift gears in my thinking and reactions to everything about me."

"I think I know what you mean," Ezra answered. "I had a devil of a time accepting the fact that my recuperation was going to be problematical. I knew I couldn't work steadily as I had before. I became bored and restless. I felt lonely, sort of like being ostracized from medicine completely. I'm a workhorse and I love being a physician and helping patients. That was my greatest pleasure in life. Now I can't be a physician anymore. I suppose I'll be able to find hobbies. Roz and I are going to buy a boat; maybe that will be a distraction. But I can't take medicine out of my mind and thinking processes."

I turned to stare at his profile as we walked. I felt both compassion and unhappiness for my dear friend. I wished I had a magic wand at that very moment. I would have waved it over him and granted his every wish.

"Well, one never knows what new developments will come over the horizon and give you back your abilities."

"Thanks," he mumbled in the wind.

He was right in his estimation of his situation. He had accepted it totally — regretfully and possibly with some anger, however.

"Well, you can always take my blood pressure," I chided him.

The days passed too quickly. As we rested in the sun, we exchanged ideas about how to help the recovering bypass patient. I suggested that perhaps he could take on a few patients, as he had done with me, to keep himself busy in medicine. He had helped me so much, how much more could he do with non-physician patients!

"I did consider doing that, but, you see, I don't have the stamina. When you sleep in the afternoon, I do the same. And remember, I had my bypass three years before yours."

"How about one patient at a time?" I asked.

"Not enough return for the time," he answered. "I'm not talking about money but about knowing that I would have to be on call. That's the problem; I don't have that capacity anymore."

"What should *I* do?" I asked.

"Give your patients reassurance and encouragement. Be firm, authoritative about their exercise and dieting, impress them with the need to avoid stress."

"And remember our genetic influences," I added.

Time passed too rapidly and soon it was the night before we had to leave. I would make copious notes about our talks, promising myself that I would do what I could for the group that had formed back home. I knew Vinnie was home, and Tony would be home by now, too. I would give my time to all members of the group and try to do for them what Ezra had done for me. I began to outline my first paper of counseling post-surgery bypass patients.

Sexual matters would be more difficult than other topics to communicate about. Perhaps it was something I felt in myself. Ezra knew how I treated sexual problems in my practice and how I taught the subject, but I could not broach the subject often with him. There was a certain propriety to him, not an aloofness, just my instinct that this kind of talk would not be appropriate. It would have to come later when working with other bypass patients. However, what I had experienced sexually was so important to me, I felt that the subject must be a compelling one for many others. For a moment I thought of the young man in Milwaukee who was so concerned about his own performance after surgery. There had to be answers and I knew in time they would come to me.

On our last night in Florida, Carol and I took Ezra and Roz out to dinner. We drank wine, ate fish and poultry, and exchanged the kind of pleasant nonsense in which friends indulge.

I truly didn't want to leave, but I had to return to Connecticut
to have my blood chemistry checked and to take my first stress
test. We said our good-byes that night for we were leaving early
in the morning. As I turned, I remember saying over my shoulder, "Goodbye old friend! I really will miss you."

"Hey, Joe," his voice called after we'd turned to leave, "If
you need your blood pressure checked, fly down and I'll do it
gratis."

I waved to him. Carol took my hand as we walked back to
the apartment. She knew what I was feeling and we walked
slowly in silence in the warm night air.

About six weeks had passed since the operation, and I was
scheduled for my first stress test. I reported to the cardiology
department of Stamford Hospital at about 8:30 in the morning.
I had been allowed no breakfast before the test. All the staff
seemed to know that I was expected; I changed into a pair of
jogging shorts. I also wore my warm socks and jogging shoes. In
the examining room I saw the treadmill; there was a large
machine before the treadmill flickering numbers and lights. It
was a mystery to me. The nurse asked me to lie on the bed,
which was on one side of the room. She attached electrodes
to my chest and I watched as she ran an EKG.

"This is the resting EKG," she explained. "Dr. Landesman
will be along soon and we'll start the stress test."

As she spoke, Richard Landesman entered smiling and
making me feel comfortable; he checked the resting EKG.
"Looks the same as those I do in the office. Now, let's begin."

I stood on the treadmill and was told to hold on to the bar
in front of me for balance. He attached the electrodes, still
pasted on my chest, to some plugs in the machine looming
ahead of me and wrapped a blood pressure cuff around my left
arm. While he was taking my blood pressure, I noticed a light
appear before me. It was a number: *84*. I was told that that was
my pulse rate. As my pressure was being taken I could see the
number constantly change to *86 — 88 — 86 — 84*.

"Now we're going to start the treadmill," Richard explained.
"It will be slow at first and we'll increase the speed as we go
along. If you feel any change, such as constriction or tightness,
or any symptom that is different from those you have become

accustomed to, let me know, please. That's your pulse rate before you. Don't concentrate on that. It signifies the amount of beats that I'd like you to reach before we stop. I'll explain more about that later. Shall we begin?"

"Contact!" I said. The treadmill moved slowly and I began to walk slowly, matching the rate of the motion beneath my feet.

I noticed that as soon as I started to walk, my pulse jumped to 98. It must be anxiety, I told myself. I had taken my pulse at home while resting and it usually registered about 70 to 80. I continued walking and noticed the continuous feed of paper was coming out of the right side of the machine. Richard studied it and then said, "We're going to increase the speed now. Just hold on to the bar for balance."

The treadmill began to move faster, and now I could see my pulse registering 106. God, I thought is it that high? Is something wrong? But as I continued to walk at the same pace, the pulse dropped to 94. Again the EKG paper was feeding out of the side of the machine. Richard studied it, and as I walked he took my blood pressure.

"We're going to increase the pace again, and this time you'll notice that the platform will tilt upwards a little."

As he spoke, I could feel the tilting and the speed increasing. My pulse was registering 114; when I walked faster, I could see my pulse stabilizing at around 106. I was beginning to feel a little tired, but I didn't say anything. Again, the EKG began to feed out of the machine; Richard glanced at it and took my blood pressure again. Then I could feel the platform tilting further upwards and the speed increasing. I kept up with the speed; my pulse was now generally reading about 136 and seemed to stay near that number. Every once in a while Richard took my pressure and glanced at the EKG paper. Again, he increased the speed; in reaction, my pulse read 148. I continued at that pace while the pressure was taken once more, and now I was beginning to breathe hard.

"Notice any change in your feelings?" Richard asked.

"Just feeling a little tired," I said, breathing hard.

"Just another minute or so." he replied. My pulse rate was now hovering in the general area of 152.

"Now we're going to slow down" Richard said. "When the treadmill stops, you may feel a little dizzy. When you get off, I'd like you to lie on the bed and rest."

The machine slowly came to a halt and I stepped off. I did feel dizzy. I walked to the bed and stretched out. I felt no pain or change in any symptoms or feelings in my chest. I watched Richard as he went through the roll of EKG tracings. Shortly he said, "It looks good, Joe." He took my blood pressure again. "I'll send a report to Dr. Kanter."

"Everything all right?" I asked.

"So I just said," he replied. "Rest there a while until the nurse lets you know when to get dressed."

"Richard," I began, "do I just keep doing the exercises and keep taking the medication?"

"Yes," he answered. "Call Dr. Kanter next week. He'll have my full report then. Dr. Kanter will be the one who will regulate your medication. How're you feeling now?"

"Great," I said. "My breathing is back to normal."

"Now when you walk, try to get your pulse rate up to the vicinity of 130 to 140. By walking faster, you'll find your pulse will reach that level. There is a simple formula to use. Subtract your age from the number 200. In your case you would subtract 55, leaving 145 as the maximum level or target that you should try to achieve. But between 130 to 140 would be acceptable. Any number in that range would determine good exercising of the heart muscle. Like any muscle, it should be worked."

He left the room and I continued to rest. The nurse who had been with us throughout the procedure remained in the room. Finally, she took my blood pressure once more, removed the cuff, and instructed me to dress. I did and drove home feeling satisfied with my progress.

When I arrived home, I related everything about the test to Carol. To celebrate, we decided to go for a brisk walk. I bundled up in my usual fashion looking like an alien from a frozen planet.

We did a brisk mile but then the wind came up, followed by a flurry of snow. Cursing at the damnable weather, we went home.

That night I called my group of friends in Connecticut and

told them the results. We were all happy for each other. Vinnie would be next at the stress-test stage, and Bob and Tony would not be far behind, depending on what their own cardiologists decided. My results encouraged them a great deal. They felt that if my results were OK, theirs also had to be OK; after all, we were all in the same boat together.

They came over that evening with their wives and we spent the evening talking about the test and a lot of other, mostly lightweight, topics. It was difficult to discuss what living with coronary disease had been like before we'd gone to the hospital. I am sure that each of us recalled his own stresses and strains, his own pain, his own anxieties, his own fears, and his own wonder at the continuation of his life. But the subject could not be discussed openly. It was like ancient history that belonged in the past, and one must look ahead to tomorrow. That was the way it was with us. At ten o'clock I looked at my watch, and announced, "Do you know, fellas, it is about an hour past my usual bedtime." They agreed that the hour was late for them, too. One of the women said she had become so accustomed to going to bed no later than 8:00 or 8:30 and getting all this rest that she never realized it was so late. I commented that ten o'clock was hardly what I would have considered late several months ago, but I did consider ten o'clock late nowadays. We said our goodbyes, and shortly, I am certain, we were all asleep.

Now as the days passed, I began to notice a certain shift in my emphases, from the physical to the psychological aspects of recovery. I arrived at no earthshaking conclusions by any means, and there was no outward change reflecting my mental state, I think, but, slowly, changes *were* beginning to occur. I would have to say that I would go through a singular experience several times as if I were testing myself, and wondering about the meaning of that particular experience. I needed time, I had to admit, to clarify and analyze what was going on inside me. The physical aspects of my recovery seemed to have come to an end in a sense (although, of course, they had not; I still had to exercise) but my *concern* over the physical aspects had ended and I had started to concentrate on my psychological well being. I had strange thoughts. Does the bypass operation affect one's longevity, I asked myself. It goes without saying that the longevity is increased, of course. I know in my particular case, had I not had the bypass operation, then ultimately that widow's artery was going to make a widow out of Carol. That was a certainty. In my mind I knew this to be so. I had no scientific evidence to dispute it, but I knew it would have happened sooner had I not had this bypass operation. Now perhaps the question of longevity is something YOU don't think about. One doesn't give it much thought when one is younger. Sometimes when I would speak to medical students or interns or residents at a hospital, I would say to myself they probably don't have a thought about longevity. It was just taken for granted. One could almost hear them saying, "Well, of course, I'm going to live forever." There was a sense of immortality in their youthfulness; there was a sense of immortality in the fact that the years passed very slowly.

One evening, as I was preparing myself to take it easy and do a little reading, I recalled a conversation with an old anatomy professor in my freshman year in medical school. He has long since gone, but I was fond of him. In our freshman year at medical school, there was a young man, who most of us felt was a charming, gregarious, pleasant person, certainly without problems, (except for the typical problem of freshman medical students — not having enough time to study). We were shocked one Monday morning to discover that this young man had locked himself in a hotel room and taken an overdose of sleeping pills. Nobody could guess his motives. Another young fellow, a particularly good friend of his, kept muttering that he didn't understand it; there was no apparent reason.

I suspect even then that I was able to analyze that one *really* does not know any other person; even in the best friendship there is only limited understanding. There is a multitude of beliefs, desires, and secrets that shape the personality; with so many variables, no two personalities are more than marginally similar. It was much later, when I became a psychiatrist, that the truth of this came to my attention; that no two patients can be treated in exactly the same way. No two people have similar secrets and experiences and desires. We all have our own hidden secrets, as it must have been for this freshman medical student. Those secrets prompted him and frightened him so that he found no other alternative to deal with his problem, but to bring his problems to an abrupt end. I remember saying to the anatomy professor that I supposed none of us could know the real reason, and he agreed with me. I made a statement that was a cliché—I recall saying it because I was embarrassed at the strong motive a fellow student must have had to do this to himself. I was embarrassed for him, for myself, and for the entire class, and I was especially embarrassed that medicine, which should have offered a method for dealing with this sort of despair, had been helpless to prolong this young man's life.

That's what I was feeling that evening as I was settling down to read: that now medicine had done something for me to prolong my life—given me a sense of longevity.

What made me think of this incident was something the professor had said to me. I repeat it, not to *prove* a particular point, but to share the understanding I achieved, that life is short.

"You know, Joe," my anatomy professor began, "this year the actuarial statistics claim that men live an average of 68.4 years, and women average 71.3 years." Although I heard him out, I could not become enthusiastic about the subject: old age seemed unreachably remote. The professor was reading my mind.

"You are 23, aren't you, Joe?"

I said, "Yes."

"It seems to you that 68.4 is a long way from now, doesn't it?" I felt embarrassed and laughed self-consciously. He must have been close to that age. "How are you in mathematics?" he asked.

I replied, "I'm afraid I'm not too good."

He reached for a piece of chalk on his desk and told me to take it to the blackboard. I obeyed and waited for instructions. He began: "Now you'll recall, we said 68 and some months. Let's even it out and say 70 years. Let's just say that men being in good health will live to 70 years. OK?"

"It's all right with me," I said.

"Let's not think of it, though, in terms of years. Let's think of it in terms of months."

"Months?" I asked.

"Yes, simply months. Now write on that blackboard. Seventy times twelve. You know, Joe, twelve months a year for seventy years. How many months is that?"

I wrote, 70 × 12 = 840 months. As I wrote the figure *840* and added the word *months*, a strange feeling came over me. Eight hundred forty months did not seem so long. Seventy years seemed a *much* longer time than 840 months.

"Now, Joe," the professor continued, "let us subtract 23 — that's what you said you were — from 70. Come on, put it up on that board."

Dutifully, I put down 70 and put 23 under it, and subtracted and got the number 47. Now the professor had joined me at the blackboard, and with his piece of chalk he wrote, "47 × 12 = 564 months."

I was amazed by those figures: there were only 564 months that I supposedly had left to reach my actuarial end. I had squandered (it seemed to me) almost 300 months already. Where had they gone?

"That's a devastating way to look at life" I remarked.

"Oh, I agree," the professor replied. "Most assuredly, I agree. Now look at me; I am 67 this month. I have only fifteen months to fill my actuarial table."

And my head spun. I thought the whole subject was repulsive; why in the world were we talking this way?

"Now you can see," the professor went on, "as medical men, although we can only take life as it comes, we never take life for granted, because we know that each patient that walks into our office has only a limited number of months to live."

I was not listening to his philosophizing about the practice of medicine. I was looking at my friend and thinking about his single year left to live. What a dreadful thought, I said to myself. "There are always exceptions," I blurted out. "We know that there are many men who live to their seventies, eighties, nineties, and some even past a hundred years old."

"That's true," he replied, "but there are many men who die at thirty or forty or fifty or sixty. Those statistics are fairly accurate, Joe. They even out: They average out. On average, a man like you has 564 months to go, Joe. Let's hope it's much longer and that in those extra months (those few hundred months) you will be a fine physician, one whom I would be proud of."

Looking at the blackboard, I said to myself that 564 months is not a very long time. The months fly by quickly. If you, reader, really want to get upset, follow my example: Take your age; deduct it from a realistic figure for a lifespan (70, 75, 80 years); then multiply the result by 12. The product is the number of months you have left. If I will live to be seventy, then I have 15 years × 12 = 180 months to live.

Remembering that incident, I recalled the many arguments pro and con about the bypass operation. There were many cardiologists who are quite certain that any sort of coronary problem can be treated with medication. It is their view that one experiences, say, angina to warn one that there is something wrong with one's heart (it is not being fed or oxygenated properly, or the blood supply is getting a little diminished.) They think that medication and medical treatment are preferable to a surgical bypass. I am sure they are sincere in what they say, and I suppose that it depends upon which artery they are discussing, but even with regard to those men who have the left coronary artery involved, I can still hear certain cardiologists say there is no need for surgical intervention—let us treat it medically.

I have a friend who suffered for fourteen years with severe angina. If the weather was cold, if he had to walk too fast, if he had to climb a hill, if he had to run, his chest felt constricted. He felt angina, I spoke to him often, especially after I had returned from my own bypass operation, and I couldn't understand why he never permitted an angiogram, why he was not being catheterized, why his arteries were not being examined so that one would know what was going on inside his chest. If there ever was a fellow who deserved a second chance, and a chance to have this pain removed, it was my friend.* I felt such fury and such anger that whoever spoke to him, or treated him, or advised him did so with the idea that those pills and medicines were going to keep him content and alive. Now they may keep him alive, but I don't think they would keep him content, and

*Since this was written, he has undergone a surgical bypass performed by Dr. Shore, and I have just been informed that he did well and is now in the Intensive Care Unit.

I don't think that he particularly enjoyed living with the constant specter of pain. As I thought about the calculation I had done for my anatomy professor, I thought of my friend. I asked myself, now that he has new vessels, how many months will he have? Certainly in my mind he had been given more months, more years.

It is only those who are truly involved — the cardiologists and the cardiac surgeons — who can establish the rules. It is a great tragedy to me to see the squabbling that one reads about in every issue of the medical journals, and it causes even newspapers to report this particular disagreement. But, you see, we physicians are a peculiar breed. We will fight, it is true, and argue, and say and do an awful lot of silly things, but in the end, there will be a good, valid, scientific answer which will help all humanity. Every man who is in good health today (and can dispense the possibility of developing severe illnesses such as cancer or diabetes), knows that the *heart* is going to be his problem as he gets older, and as each month passes by, that is what he must save and protect.

Fifteen

Learning from Each Other

Gradually, a sizable group of bypass veterans was formed. We met at each other's homes and just talked about our problems. The group was inclined to talk freely about various physical problems, forgetting that I was a psychiatrist rather than a cardiologist. It interested me that most of the men were very concerned about their sexual performance. I encouraged them to trust their own emotions and desires. I offered no advice, as a sexual therapist might do ordinarily; I thought that it was important that each patient find his own way. Whenever a problem arose, inevitably it was my phone that rang and one of the men would ask to speak to me privately. At such times I offered some advice, telling about studies that had shown that the energy used in climbing several flights of stairs was more than the amount required for intercourse. One had to judge his own capabilities.

In time, I felt impelled to write about the experiences of the eight members of the group. I belong to New York Medical College Department of Sexual Therapy. The department was under the aegis of Virginia Sadock, M.D., with whom I had trained. My supervisor was Jacquiline Hott, Ph.D. One evening when we met in New York, I related my talks with the bypass group. Dr. Sadock suggested that perhaps I could write a medical article describing my experiences with the group. Dr. Hott also encouraged me to write and suggested that when the manuscript was finished, she would like to get it published in a scholarly journal called *Sexuality and Disability*. She was on the editorial board and felt the article would be an interesting contribution. The problem is widespread: Each year more than 100,000 bypass operations are performed in this country. The response to the article in *Sexuality and Disability* was enormous. I received requests for reprints from all over the country and throughout the world. It astounded me that after all these years no one had dealt before with what I considered a very serious aspect of bypass surgery.

I presented the paper at the annual meeting of the American Association for Sex Therapy and Research. It was during this meeting I found that many other therapists were confronted by the problems I had elucidated in my paper. Soon I was talking to various groups throughout the area, and my own group expanded to twenty-six members. As members improved physically and psychologically, they left, and new ones joined the group.

In the beginning we seemed to flounder around, simply reassuring each other as Ezra had reassured me. Gradually, we became more sophisticated in offering support. For example, I noticed that each time the weather changed, I developed an itch along the suture line down my sternum. I thought nothing of it, however. At one of our meetings, when I found myself scratching my chest, I noticed two others doing the same.

"Is anyone itching?" I asked.

"I feel that way when the weather changes," one of the men answered.

"So do I," added the second patient.

We started to laugh and all of us began to itch. Some admitted that they had been unaware of the feeling until the subject had been brought up.

"What causes that? I never itch," stated one man.

"Just a guess on my part." I answered. "Those wires they use to sew up the sternum must expand and contract in some miniscule way, and the tightening and loosening of those wires may be the culprit."

"What a relief!" one of the scratchers said. "I was afraid that it was a twinge of angina, yet it wasn't like any angina I had in the past."

I related to the group that it had made me so apprehensive that I had asked my cardiologist to check it out. I never had angina that I knew of, but I thought that this might have been the start of it. One of the other "itchers" confided that he had done the same, but no one had explained about the wires before.

"That's only a guess," I said. "But it seems to be possibly true. I am aware of this each time the weather changes. The itch has always coincided with a drop in the barometer and I would know that the next day it would snow or rain. So I guess tomorrow will not be as sunny as today."

The phone rang three times at my home the next morning. It was a snowy, windy day, with the snow piling up almost a foot and with drifts of up to two feet outside my window. All the callers were joking about our "barometer."

On February 13, 1981, I was busy in the library at St. Joseph's Hospital when I felt that my chest began itching. The itch seemed excessively irritating. I knew from the morning paper that the weather was to be sunny and fair for the next three days. I continued to work, mumbling to myself that the weatherman was wrong again. I finished the work in the library in the afternoon and returned home. When I walked into the house, I mentioned my itch to Carol and told her that it would probably rain or snow tomorrow.

"That's interesting," Carol said. "Usually you get that itch when the barometer falls, but I have some news for you. The radio just announced that the barometer has hit an extremely high reading; that it went so high that the reading went off the barometric machine the weather people use." Sure enough, the following morning the *New York Times* reported that the barometer reading reached the highest level in more than fifty years. I was a walking barometer!

I called several others in the group; they had the same experience as I. Any time you want to know about barometric pressure, just ask your friendly bypass patient.

Other oddities appeared. Vinnie one time mentioned that while driving he would develop moderate pain in his thigh where it rested on the edge of the car seat. (The saphenous vein had been removed in that leg from the ankle to the groin.) Many men agreed. The symptom continued for over a year. Many suggestions were offered for overcoming the difficulty. One day Vinnie stated that he'd found the solution. He placed a fluffy pillow on the car seat, raising his body a few inches; in this way he relieved the pressure on his thigh. Since it was on his right side, (the foot used on the accelerator), it made the discomfort more tolerable. One fellow ingeniously formed a foam rubber pillow that supported his leg at the edge of the car seat. He made a few more for other fellow sufferers.

In the beginning of our meetings, wives were excluded from the group. But an incident changed our collective thinking. A patient had been extremely apprehensive about sexual relations. The desire was there, but because of his anxiety he needed a nitroglycerine tablet prior to intercourse. He did not have angina any more, so he wondered whether he should take the nitro.

"Why take it if you don't have angina?" asked another member.

"I don't know. Habit, maybe. I thought I would feel safer."

"Don't do it," another said. "Try first, and see what happens."

"I agree," another added. "I feel apprehensive, too. I tried once but I was unable to perform. I know I'm not impotent because I often wake with erections. If you succeed, then I'll try it again." He pointed to another in the group. "It's a serious problem with me and him. We discussed it one day while exercising. There has to be some solution."

I reported my own experience, but it was not considered relevant, because I had never had angina.

Another man offered his experience instead. I knew him quite well because he had come to my office to try to overcome a great amount of anxiety he experienced. A few reassuring sessions were all he needed. I recall his story as he related it.

"I saw Joe in his office a few times because of this problem," he began. "Joe gave me a few tablets of Ativan. How do you describe that tablet?"

"It's an antianxiety medication," I responded, "very mild."

"That's it. Joe suggested it would melt if I placed it under my tongue, just as my nitro did. Well, fellas, it worked like a charm. I was successful—no angina. I used it four times. Joe said it was no longer necessary after that—I was using it like a crutch. I tried getting by without it and since then had no problems. I think I needed that crutch for a little while."

"Can I get a prescription?" asked another in the group.

"No," I replied. "You just heard him admit that it's a crutch. It's no help having to depend on a crutch."

The following meeting three of the men reported that they no longer had anxiety about love making. But one member made an interesting observation.

"When I started to make love to my wife, I sensed she was very tense and she kept asking if I felt all right. Her questions annoyed me and it made me wonder if she was correct in her concern. I found myself reassuring her. Which leads me to ask this question for the group: Do you think it would help to have our wives here when we meet? It would reassure them, too. I think my wife was much more apprehensive about intercourse than I was. What do you guys think?"

At the following meeting a considerable number of wives joined us. I felt that this was the most important step the group made, to include the wives in some of the meetings. Our first female member was accompanied by her husband. One of the men began to ask her about her sexual life and had great difficulty in getting his question out. An astute, sensitive person, she quickly surmised what he was leading up to in his roundabout manner of questioning.

"I feel better knowing there are other women in this meeting," she began. "I, too, felt the same as you men. Perhaps a trifle different. I felt self-conscious about the scar between my breasts and thought it would be a turn-off for my husband." At this point her husband reached over and held her hand. "He was wonderful about it. Just touching the scar, running his hand along it, made me feel so much better. I felt he still wanted me." In a softer tone of voice she added, "He still desired me."

The wives of the male patients began to applaud spontaneously.

"Can I ask a question?" one of the wives asked. "I'm glad I'm here. You men think only about your own feelings. I would like to share my feelings, if I may." She hesitated a moment, looking about her, and then, feeling there was support (it was unverbalized, but perhaps she saw something in the faces and eyes of the other women), she continued. "I think I can talk for the other wives here. I, too, was very apprehensive when we first made love. God, I thought to myself, suppose — suppose something goes wrong? I was just as apprehensive as my husband. Maybe more so. I apologize if I sound competitive as to who felt more anxiety, but I know I was tense and nervous, too. You can't imagine the relief I felt when it was over. It sounds terrible, but I felt no enjoyment at the time. My joy was in knowing my husband had overcome a frightening, deadly hurdle. For that, I was happiest." Then she laughed and added, "It's been great ever since."

The group all joined in, laughing and making jokes directed at the speaker's husband. It was delightfully Rabelaisian.

"My turn," a new member called above the noise of the group. He had been operated on only three weeks ago, and as he spoke he was still short of breath; often had to rest and breathe deeply before he could speak. I marveled at the patience of the entire group; we were all genuinely supportive. "I've learned a great deal here today. Your discussion, I hope, will help me later on, maybe sooner than I can imagine. I've noticed something about myself I don't like." He was breathing very heavily now, and he spoke more slowly as the group directed its full attention to him. "I'm irritable with myself and everyone else. I feel like a damn baby. I have to be helped up the stairs sometimes. I even have to be helped to dress. I feel helpless, dependent. It's not me. I ran a large corporation. I was quick in my decisions, alert to problems, and capable of dealing daily with a countless number of people. Now I don't want anyone around. I feel depressed and I hate this constant dependency that permeates everything I do or think. I insist that my wife walk with me when I exercise. I'm afraid I'll just drop dead in the middle of a step. This is not me. I'm someone else. A cripple. Worst of all, I feel ashamed of what I feel."

The group was silent. One could feel the welling up of a wave of empathy, zeroing in on this new member.

"Perhaps I can help." one of our older group members offered. "I'm the president of a large international chemical-manufacturing corporation. What you just told us, I also experienced. I wouldn't answer the phone at home for fear it was my secretary calling for a decision I had to make. My wife would just say I was sleeping; it was a lie, of course, but I couldn't and didn't want to speak to anyone. Even talking was an effort."

I looked towards the first man who had spoken to determine his reaction. The man talking was in his league as an executive in a large corporation; they had something essential in common. He was listening intently; the jiggling foot was no longer moving. He was breathing slowly and evenly. The second man had gotten through to him.

"So patience is something we all had to learn and you will, too," the second executive concluded. When the meeting had ended, the two men arranged to meet for further discussion and exercise. Three years later I heard that their companies had merged.

One day while at home I received a call from a member of the group named Frank. He was always quiet and seemed shy about talking in the group. He wanted to see me in my office. I was working only a few hours a day, two days a week. I suggested that he meet on a day when I wasn't working so that I wouldn't be influenced by the clock and we could spend as much time together as was necessary.

"I've had a problem all my life," Frank said. "I guess I'm what you would call a premature ejaculator. It always bothered me, but it didn't seem to make much difference to my wife. She's a good woman, but I don't think she ever enjoyed sex. It's very hard talking about something so intimate, you know, so personal. I thought that after the operation I would slow down and have more staying power. It isn't happening. My wife keeps saying it's O.K., but it's not O.K. with me."

I explained that sexual therapy for him and his wife could probably help the situation to their mutual satisfaction. I explained that since I knew him socially I could not treat them, but I suggested that they see someone in New York where he worked. He and his wife could make a weekly holiday out of the day he met with the therapist.

About six months later, I learned that Frank's experience in sexual therapy was successful. It was Frank who brought the subject up when another member made a comment about persistent impotence. Frank took the floor and described his treatment. His wife told the women in the group about her reaction when she had learned to be orgasmic for the first time in her life. That entire meeting was a lecture given by Frank and his wife about the possibility to change, if one wanted it, and about seeking help for sexual problems.

"One thing I've learned," Frank said, "is that if you have a problem before bypass, it won't change after the operation. I can't imagine how anyone could think otherwise."

I had to admit our group really was becoming a sophisticated, cohesive, nice bunch of men and women. I was very proud of them. Sexuality was comfortably discussed, and this attitude was passed on to new members. All patients were indoctrinated with this attitude when they joined.

Another source of anxiety was taking the first stress test. It usually was given about six to eight weeks after the patient returned home. Since I had already gone through the test, I described it to the group. When Vinnie had to have his stress test, he asked me to come along with him. I met him at St Joseph's Hospital where his cardiologist, Dr. Yap, put him through his paces. I think the fact that I was in the room with him, even though I said nothing, helped him relax and go through the test with less anxiety. As a rule, one experienced member of the group would join a newer member for his first stress test. It was good to see the friendly face of someone who had already been through the same experience. The patient's dependency and passivity of the early recuperative stages typically was overcome after the first stress test. Once reassured by the cardiologist that all was well and that there were no signs of angina, the patient quickly resumed his presurgical behavior.

However, a new pattern of behavior became apparent during the second and third years following surgery. Three men obtained a divorce; the choice was theirs. I found an interesting reaction in these men. These men had never considered the relationships with their wives significant. They became involved with other women who seemed to provide more warmth and less stress in their interpersonal lives. At first the group reacted in a negative fashion. Most of us desired to keep the status quo in our marital relationships. There were attempts at convincing the men to reconsider their action. Only one member would discuss the subject openly in the group. He was very convincing, emphasizing his need for tranquility and a less stressful relationship, and he won the group over. Nothing more was said about the subject. The group continued with the meetings and self-help for each other.

Meanwhile I had received a call from Don Kanter's office to come in for a follow-up and discussion of the stress test. Carol and I went to see him. He drew some blood for further blood chemistry, did a thorough physical examination, and then told us that the stress test had been excellent. He urged continuation of the exercises, but then he said, "I see no reason for you to continue taking any more medication. Let's stop all pills. Just take a multivitamin in the morning." He closed the folder. "Any questions?"

I was so pleased and thankful that I could stop all medication, I was speechless. I shook my head and Carol thanked him for his genuine concern and good care.

"Once a year you are to call Dr. Landesman for another stress test. Before the test is made, have a complete blood chemistry done at the hospital laboratory. Make certain that you request a lipid study so that we can follow your cholesterol levels as well as the triglycerides and the HDL studies. If you suspect any symptoms, don't hesitate to let me know."

"What's HDL?" I asked. "I think I remember George Walcott saying something about this to me at St. Mary's Hospital after the operation. I guess I forgot."

"High-density lipoprotein. It simply means a different kind of fat in your blood stream. It's a good kind. It doesn't deposit in the lining of those coronary arteries but rather it seems to pull the cholesterol crystals out of one's blood stream. If your HDL is high, that's a good sign. Yours is about 30 now. I would like to see it move up with exercise and diet."

"I'm really getting to be an obsessive-compulsive. I take the smallest piece of chicken skin and peel it away."

Don laughed. "Look, there's no need for that! Every once in awhile you can go off the diet. I repeat, only once in awhile. The most important aspect of your recovery is without a doubt exercise and more exercise. Do that and it will make me happy and you healthier. Agreed?"

"Agreed," I answered.

We shook hands, although I wanted to hug him. Instead Carol gave him a hug and a kiss and we left the office.

The winter was still ravaging Connecticut with freezing temperatures and violent snow storms. I needed to find an indoor location for my exercises. The local YMCA was too crowded; I needed a place with less noise and interference with my walking. I finally found the perfect place, the Spartan Club; it is affiliated with the Greek church in town. I drove down to the club and met Gus K. Since I could not pronounce his last name we both agreed to call him Gus. Gus was a retired school principal in his sixties. He was in excellent physical health, and I admired his tenacity in racquet-ball playing. He swam and worked out and exercised hard every day. The first day he showed me the large basketball gym and explained that walking twenty times around the perimeter was equal to one mile. There was a regulation-size swimming pool; thirty-six laps equal to a mile. There were two racquet-ball courts, and there was a large room with an international gym, weights for lifting and strengthening the arms and chest muscles, a stationary bicycle, rowing machines, and more. This was for me; I joined. The membership was kept small deliberately, kept that way to avoid overcrowding and conflicting activities.

When I explained to Gus the reasons I chose the Spartan Club, he informed me that there were several men who had had bypass surgery and that I probably would meet them.

Downstairs, there was a large locker room, the showers, a large whirlpool tub, the sauna, and the steam room. I could not have asked for better facilities.

I worked out five or six times a week. The first week, climbing the stairs from the locker room to the swimming pool was exhausting. I breathed deeply until I had caught my breath and there was Gus sitting and reading while I did a slow breast stroke to strengthen my arms and chest muscles. As the weeks passed, I could recognize my own improvement. It was most gratifying.

Gus hovered over me at the club. His attention made me feel comfortable and, in a sense, protected. If anything should happen to me, he was right beside me, ready to assist in any way he could. I swam, he would sit on the edge of the pool and read, not saying a word, just keeping an eye on me. When I walked around the basketball court, he would watch from the bleacher seats until I was finished. He became a great source of comfort and reassurance as I increased the time and amount of exercise. As you see, Gus was great in my eyes.

At the beginning of March I was itching to return to work. I called Don, who reported that my blood tests were fine and that I could return to work if I limited my hours at first; as I felt more energetic I was to use my own discretion in deciding the number of hours I could put in at the office. By the end of March I was working three days a week, about five hours a day. The weather was still cold and snowy.

One day I received a call from Carol's cousin, Bluma Nathan, from Palm Beach.

"When are you coming down to stay with me?" she asked. "The weather is marvelous, the ocean inviting, and the sun will tan your hospital pallor. When can I expect you?"

I laughed at her enthusiastic invitation. "How can I refuse such graciousness?"

"Then it's settled! I'll expect you next week, Put Carol on the phone and she can explain about any special diet you may need." Carol took the phone and gave her the information she requested. A week later I was in Palm Beach. I had forgotten how comforting and relaxing the warmth of the sun could make me feel. It seemed that for the first time since the operation I did not feel chilled. Playing golf with some old friends spending the winter down there, I felt apprehensive as I teed up on the first hole. Schlossey, one friend, was standing to the side as he had done when we had played together hundreds of times.

"I think if I take a real swing at the ball," I said, "my chest will open and I'll just split in two right here."

"There's nothing like finding out," Schlossey replied. I swung at the ball and it careened down the fairway. "Not bad," Schlossey said. "How about ten cents a hole?"

"You're on," I said. I felt great. I didn't eviscerate through my suture line down my sternum and I felt good as we walked together toward our next shot. The warm weather and sun were doing their job. Energy was returning steadily. I was peaceful, stressless, and content.

Meanwhile Bluma had arranged her own schedule. She was a fine artist and often painted during the day. While I took my nap, she worked without making a sound. After dinner we would talk, but she knew that I usually retired at nine. She accommodated me by doing the same. I rested, exercised by walking several miles each morning, read on the terrace, and swam in the pool after lunch.

When I returned to Connecticut I was feeling great; I could feel the change in me. I continued to work with the group and occasionally would speak to groups that met at the New Canaan YMCA in a rehabilitation program for cardiac patients as well as bypass patients. It was good for all of us to exchange our reactions to surgery. Since I was the "elder" in terms of surgery, it reassured these men. In essence, it was mutually helpful.

Occasionally, I would get a call from someone who had heard about the group. I would then go to his home and try to answer his questions. The group was becoming quite large, so we broke into smaller, less cumbersome groups. There never was a leader. Occasionally we invited a dietician to speak to us; at other times a physiotherapist, to talk about exercising; a cardiologist; and one time a biochemist, to interpret the importance of cholesterol and lipid or fatty blood substances in our blood stream. Education was a necessity for reassurance and peace of mind.

By the end of the first year my new routine was a way of life. I worked until late afternoon only three days a week. I did not want to overwork, considering my physical limits. I exercised five or six times a week. I began jogging near the end of the first year. In the beginning I did a quarter of a mile; it took until the second year before I had enough stamina to reach a mile of jogging followed by a mile of brisk fast-paced walking around the basketball court.

Once a year I had a stress test and the results showed the success of the workouts. My blood pressure remained stabilized at 120 over 80, which is as normal as apple pie.

It is now the end of my third year. I have just completed my stress test and have been told that it was excellent. My blood chemistry shows that I am keeping my cholesterol levels and triglycerides low, and the high-density lipoprotein is beginning to approach an acceptable level, even though this level is influenced strongly by my own genetic background.

Obviously, by following the rules of bypass recuperation, one can change life-threatening forces into life-extending forces. These changes are not a matter of luck, but a matter of consistent adherence to the several changes in dieting, exercise, and avoidance of stress.

Often I have wondered in these past two years about the changes I have made in my lifestyle since I had the bypasses. Could it have been possible to avoid this coronary artery disease if I had followed the manner of living that I do today? No one can answer that. But as I continue to gain more knowledge about coronary artery disease, I begin to believe that there was a possibility for avoiding my problems if I had followed the simple procedures of living moderately.

I have already discussed this in detail with my two children. I told them frankly, they have a poor genetic background. Not only did their father have coronary artery disease, but their grandfathers, both Carol's and mine, died of coronary artery disease. Nothing can change their heredity. But individually, they can follow the principles of living that I had assumed after my bypass operation.

Now there is no smoking for them. They follow the same diet as I. Exercise has become a ritualistic form of behavior for all of us. The crisis I had to go through has made it more imperative that they not have to go through a similar crisis.

This new way of life has made a crusader out of me. I urge all of my friends to learn and benefit from my experience. Interestingly, most of my friends have done what I have asked them to do.

I urge you to do the same.